Dr Allan St John Dixon is currently Chairman of The National Osteoporosis Society. A widely respected authority on the disease, he is also Consultant Physician at the Royal National Hospital for Rheumatic Diseases in Bath.

Dr Anthony Woolf is consultant Rheumatologist at the Royal Cornwall Hospital in Truro. He is Treasurer of the National Osteoporosis Society, and was previously working at the Royal National Hospital for Rheumatic Diseases in Bath.

O P T I M A

AVOIDING OSTEOPOROSIS

Dr Allan Dixon
& Dr Anthony Woolf

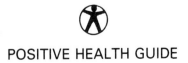

POSITIVE HEALTH GUIDE

First published in 1989 by
Macdonald Optima, a division of
Macdonald & Co. (Publishers) Ltd

A member of Maxwell Pergamon Publishing Corporation plc

British Library Cataloguing in Publication Data
Dixon, Allan St. J. (Allan St. John)
   Avoiding osteoporosis.
   1. Bones. Osteoporosis
   I. Title II. Woolf, Anthony III. Series
   616.7'1

   ISBN 0-356-15445-9

Macdonald & Co. (Publishers) Ltd
66–73 Shoe Lane
London EC4P 4AB

Photoset in Times by
🅰 Tek Art Ltd, Croydon, Surrey

**Printed and bound in Great Britain by
Mackays of Chatham PLC, Letchworth**

CONTENTS

ACKNOWLEDGEMENTS

We wish to thank Anne Davidson MCSP for preparing the exercise programmes, and Hilary Woolf for help with preparing the manuscript.

The publishers would like to thank Schering Health Care and Ciba-Geigy; Joanna Cameron for the illustrations; and Zefa.

1

WHAT IS OSTEOPOROSIS?

Osteoporosis is not a new problem. Osteoporotic bones have been found in neolithic tombs 3,000 years old. However, it has been described as the forgotten disease of the modern Western World. We are now becoming increasingly aware of it as other diseases are conquered and more of us survive into old age.

As we get older our bones break more easily, sometimes after just a trivial fall. This increased fragility of bone is what is meant by osteoporosis.

The word comes from the Greek 'osteo' for bone and porous describing the structure of the bone. Bone may appear solid, but in fact all bones are porous like a sponge. They have to be. Bones are living structures containing living cells, which have a blood supply with channels throughout the bone. Bones would be very heavy if they were solid all through, but the sponge-like structure of bone gives the maximum strength with the minimum of weight – the engineers' ideal. With age our bones become more porous than they were when young. They appear less dense on X-ray and they lose strength. Just as there can be kidney failure, heart failure or liver failure, so there is 'bone failure', and as a result an osteoporotic bone can easily fracture or crush.

The bones which most often fracture are the wrist, the hip and the vertebrae in the spine. Fracture of the wrist, known in medicine as a Colles' fracture, is a painful nuisance but not a tragedy. Fractures of the vertebrae lead to loss of height and a stoop, but fractures of the hip bone are always serious. They can result in loss of independence, and in the very elderly they can be fatal. In some regions of Britain almost one in every four elderly people who fracture a hip will die within a short

1

while, and even in the best areas the death rate is one in eight. Death is caused by the shock brought on by the injury, or by pneumonia brought on by lying on the floor for many hours awaiting help.

People with hip fractures fill many hospital beds and they cost the health service vast sums each year. They block beds which might have been available for other necessary operations such as hip-replacement surgery. In 1986 20 per cent of all orthopaedic and geriatric beds in England were filled by patients with hip fractures, and the figure is probably higher now. Vertebral fractures are a major cause of suffering, resulting in pain, loss of height, development of an unsightly stoop and the indignity of being unable to hold one's head high.

Osteoporosis is very common. We all lose some bone as we age, irrespective of sex, race or occupation. Women at all ages have less bone than men; over the age of 60 one in every four women can expect to get a fracture of some sort, but only one in 40 men.

In osteoporosis, then, the skeleton is weak, but it is usually some minor injury which finally causes a fracture. The elderly fall more often and for a variety of reasons – they may be unsteady because they have been prescribed sleeping tablets, or tablets to reduce blood pressure, they may have arthritis, a mild stroke, 'blackouts' or failing eyesight. Then, when they do fall, they fall heavily – slow reflexes and weak muscles make a hard landing more likely.

There are many factors which contribute to the loss of bone with age and there may never be any single cure for all kinds of osteoporosis. But many causes are preventable and much can be done for those who already have the condition. But let us be clear – drugs are not the whole answer. The prevention and treatment of osteoporosis does not just come out of a bottle of tablets.

This book is for those who wish to know more about this condition, either sufferers who already have osteoporosis or young women who want to avoid it. We explain the structure and working of the skeleton. We point out who is more likely to develop osteoporosis, what the problems related to it are, how to prevent it, and how to treat and cope with it if it has already happened. We answer the questions people most commonly ask, drawing on letters sent to the National Osteoporosis Society.

2

THE STRUCTURE AND PHYSIOLOGY OF BONE

The evolutionary development of a bony skeleton has taken us from the world of the slug and the worm to that of the vertebrates – large mobile creatures with highly developed but vulnerable internal organs. The skeleton gives the body its shape and supports its weight; it protects the heart and lung inside the chest, and the brain inside the skull; and it makes movement possible, operating as levers on which the muscles can act.

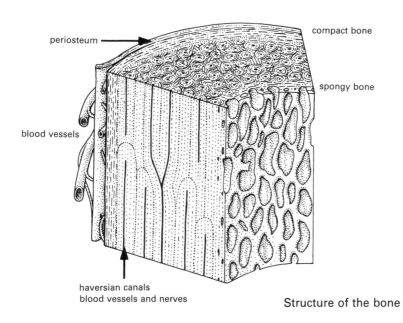

periosteum

compact bone

spongy bone

blood vessels

haversian canals
blood vessels and nerves

Structure of the bone

Bone is composed of a mineral made from calcium and phosphate, embedded in a meshwork of fibres of a protein called collagen. If it were made of mineral alone, without the collagen fibres, it would be like a piece of blackboard chalk – it would be so brittle that it would break or crumble if twisted or stretched. As an analogy, the strength of concrete is increased if the concrete is reinforced with steel rods. The comparison with reinforced concrete should not be taken too far, though, for there is an important difference – bone is a living structure.

Once it is fully developed, the skeleton is not just a sort of coat-hanger on which all the interesting bits are hung and which remains intact until it disintegrates in old age. It is continually changing, being built up and broken down by the bone cells that it contains. By the time you finish this book you will not have exactly the same skeleton that you had at the start.

STRUCTURE OF BONE

Bones are of two sorts, tubular bones and flat bones.

Tubular bones

The long bones or tubular bones are characteristically the bones of the limbs, such as the thigh bone or femur. They are the bones that bear the weight of the body.

If you cut across a long bone, you will see that it is like a hollow tube, hard and dense on the outside, the cortex, and relatively empty in the middle, the medulla. In life this space in the medulla is filled with fat.

At the ends of these long bones are joints, where the structure of the bone changes. The cortex becomes thinner and the central medulla contains a lot of criss-cross strands of bone, giving a spongy appearance and known as trabecular bone. Within this meshwork of bone lies the bone marrow – the tissue that makes blood cells.

The bones of the spine are really shortened tubular bones, with spikes and struts protruding from them which act as levers for the powerful muscles which work on the spine and keep the body upright.

This structure of the tubular bones combines maximum

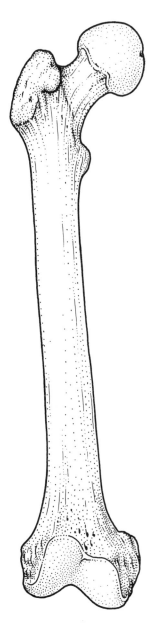

Right femur

strength, to resist compression, twisting and bending, with minimum weight.

Flat bones
The flat bones are found in the pelvis, the shoulder blades and the skull. They have a thin sandwich of medulla between two layers of cortex.

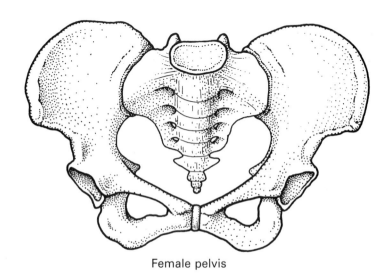

Female pelvis

COMPOSITION OF BONE

Bone, whether dense cortical bone or spongy trabecular bone, is composed of a meshwork of collagen fibres and mineral, in which calcium plays a major part.

Bone matrix
A protein called collagen forms more than a quarter of bone. The word collagen means 'jelly making'; this is because collagen, when boiled in water, breaks down to form a kind of jelly or glue. However, in their natural condition the fibres of collagen are exceedingly strong. Collagen is also found in other parts of the body and in almost all living creatures; for

example, it gives strength to the tendons that attach muscles to bones, and it is collagen that fixes shellfish such as mussels on to rocks.

There are other proteins in bone, in smaller amounts. Some have recently been discovered that appear to act as a glue to keep the minute crystals of bone mineral attached to the long tough fibres of collagen in the bone.

Bone mineral

The mineral in bone is called hydroxyapatite – a long word, but hydroxyapatite merely consists of calcium, phosphate and water. It is found as crystals attached to the collagen fibres, and its deposition in newly formed bone is known as mineralisation. Other elements found in bone, although only in minute amounts, are essential to its function, and include magnesium and fluorine.

CALCIUM

Calcium is one of the most common elements on the surface of the earth; it is the main element in limestone, chalk and marble; and almost all of it was originally part of some life form, some living organism. Whether we look at the chalk cliffs of Dover or the limestone mountains of the Alps, they were all at one time the skeletons of minute sea creatures which fell to the bottom of the sea as a mud and then became hardened and consolidated and raised up as the hills and mountains. Calcium in limestone is in the form of calcium carbonate, while calcium in the bones is a form of calcium phosphate.

If you could extract all the calcium in the body it would amount to about a kilogram (nearly 2½ pounds), 99.9 per cent of which would come from the bones. Calcium in solution, dissolved calcium, is essential for the functioning of all living cells in the body, and the concentration of this dissolved calcium in the blood is very carefully regulated. Only about 1 gram of calcium is dissolved in the blood and the rest of the body fluids; if the amount of dissolved calcium falls below this level, then more calcium is released from the bones.

The calcium we eat comes mainly from milk and cheese, from green vegetables and, in hard-water districts, from the water supply. Not all the calcium in the diet is absorbed; about two-thirds passes straight through into the faeces. However, about one-third gets through the wall of the gut into the bloodstream and then whatever is not needed for body processes or for building bones comes out in the urine. There is also some loss of calcium from the bloodstream into the intestinal juices, and this also passes into the faeces. The level of calcium in the blood, its deposition in or removal from bone, its absorption from the gut and its excretion by the kidneys into the urine are all carefully controlled by chemical messengers – hormones – discussed below.

Doctors now talk about a 'calcium balance'; that is, they measure all the calcium that goes into the body in the diet and all the calcium which comes out of the body in the urine and faeces. If more is going in than is coming out, then the difference must be deposited somewhere in the body, such as in the bones. However, a much more common situation is that more is lost from the body then goes into it; this is known as a negative calcium balance. Since the amount of calcium in the bloodstream is tightly controlled by the body, and never allowed to vary, the loss of calcium must come from the bones. And this is what happens in osteoporosis.

BONE CELLS

Osteoblasts and osteoclasts

The active cells in the bone are of two main types. There are osteoblasts, which are continually building up new bone and strengthening it. In contrast, cells called osteoclasts are responsible for the removal of bone; first they dissolve the mineral out of the bone, and this then allows the subsequent breakdown of the collagen matrix.

Under stable conditions, the amount of bone being made exactly balances the amount being removed. This continual exchange of bone is important as it allows the body to renew weakened or damaged parts of the bone, it allows for the repair of fractures, and it enables the bone to become stronger or weaker in response to how much it is used.

The balance between the formation and the removal, or resorption, of bone decides how fast the bone grows in youth, and whether it gets stronger or weaker in adult life. The rates

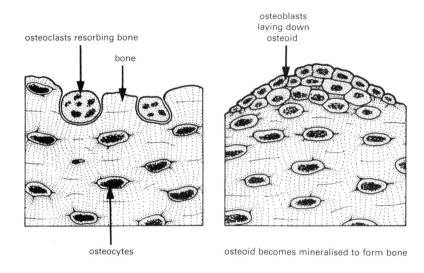

osteoclasts resorbing bone

bone

osteoblasts laying down osteoid

osteocytes

osteoid becomes mineralised to form bone

Active cells in the bone

of formation and removal of bone are normally very carefully balanced in adulthood so that, despite much turnover of bone, there is no overall loss or gain. The control of this must be very precise but is not yet fully understood.

If the osteoblasts become lazy or the osteoclasts become over-zealous then bone will be lost and osteoporosis will arise. In this case the control will have gone astray.

Osteocytes

In addition to the osteoblasts and osteoclasts, there are other cells called osteocytes. These are either embedded within bone or lie on its surface. They appear to be important in detecting and responding to local stresses applied to bone, and to the shifts of calcium between bone and blood.

DEVELOPMENT OF THE SKELETON

The foetus, childhood and growth

The framework of the skeleton develops in the foetus early in pregnancy; the long bones, for example, have their future shape and proportions by the sixth month.

9

At first the skeleton is made of softer cartilage (gristle), not bone. As it develops, though, the future skeleton becomes mineralised, and at birth the newborn baby's bones contain 25 grams (less than an ounce) of calcium. This calcium will have come from the mother's diet or, if her diet is inadequate, from her bones.

The bones of the child continue to grow during the next 20 years, with a spurt during adolescence. The growth in length of the long bones occurs near their ends, in bands known as the epiphyses; these bands can be easily seen in a child's X-ray, showing up as lighter areas. These epiphyses disappear when growth stops. The growth in the width of the long bones occurs by removal of bone from the inside of the tube and its formation on the outside.

Consolidation

Once the bones have reached their maximum size, by the age of 16–18 in girls and 18–20 in boys, they fill out, becoming denser and stronger as more mineral is laid down. This is known as the period of consolidation.

Loss

It is during these periods of growth and consolidation that we lay down our bone 'stock', and it is from this 'stock' that bone is lost as we age.

After the age of about 35–40 years, bone loses mineral very gradually. The loss can be measured using special machines. If bones are well made in our youth they should last us into old age, and even if the bone stock is not as good as it should be it will be many years before the skeleton runs into trouble.

Women, however, have an additional problem. They have an acceleration in the rate of loss of bone, starting just before and continuing for several years – probably about 10 years – after the menopause. From then on bone continues to be lost at about the original rate. Men do not have this problem. They lose bone at a steady rate from about 40 years onwards, without a 'male menopause' effect.

Women have less bone than men throughout life anyhow but, because of this additional menopause-associated loss, the difference between men and women becomes much more marked in the elderly, and explains why women are ten times more likely to fracture their bones in later life.

Gain and loss of bone in average men and women with advancing age

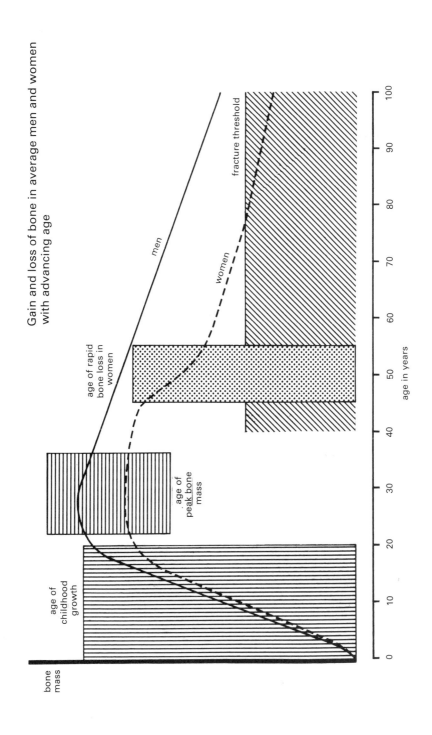

bone mass

age of childhood growth

age of peak bone mass

age of rapid bone loss in women

men

women

fracture threshold

age in years

HORMONES WHICH AFFECT BONE

The growth of bone, its mineralisation, its continual formation and resorption, its repair after fracture, its response to stresses are all under the control of chemical messengers within the body – the hormones. Some of these hormones affect the skeleton as a whole, but there are also local hormones made in the bones, produced by one cell to act on its near neighbours, co-ordinating their activities.

Parathyroid hormone, calcitonin and vitamin D are the main controlling influences on the calcium in the body. However, there are other important hormones which affect the strength of the skeleton – the sex hormones and the adrenal hormones.

Parathyroid hormone and calcitonin

These are the two important hormones that act on bone. Both are made in glands that are not directly linked to the skeleton; parathyroid hormone is made in small glands – the parathyroid glands – behind the thyroid gland in the neck while calcitonin is made in the thyroid gland itself.

Between them parathyroid hormone and calcitonin maintain the amount of calcium in the blood at a constant level. If the level falls too low, extra parathyroid hormone is made. This stimulates the osteoclasts which invade and dissolve bone, mobilising more calcium. Parathyroid hormone also acts on the kidneys, reducing the loss of calcium in the urine and on the gut, increasing the absorption of calcium from the food. Conversely, if the level of calcium in the blood becomes too high then more calcitonin is made, which shuts down the osteoclasts and stops them dissolving bone.

Vitamin D

Another hormone that has an important effect on the skeleton is vitamin D. Most vitamin D is made by the action of ultraviolet rays in sunlight on fatty materials in the skin but some is taken in in the diet, largely in fish oils. It is also added artificially to many foodstuffs, especially margarines.

Its main effect is on the gut, where it increases the absorption of calcium from the food. It is also important for the normal formation of bone. Without it, new bone that is made is not properly mineralised. This condition is called rickets in children and osteomalacia in adults. The poorly mineralised bones that result are weak, do not grow properly and develop cracks which are painful and do not heal properly.

Sex hormones

The sex hormones, called oestrogens in women and androgens in men, have their major effects on what are called the secondary sex characteristics – the development of the beard in men, and the breasts in women, as well as on the growth at puberty of the genital organs in both sexes. But this is not the only function of these hormones. They help to maintain the activity and health of all cells in the body – skin, muscles, bone and circulation are all affected by them.

Sex hormones probably work on bone cells by allowing them to respond fully to the other major controlling hormones – parathyroid hormone, calcitonin and vitamin D. At any rate, they are necessary for full bone-cell health; without them bones become more osteoporotic, particularly in women.

Female sex hormones (oestrogens) are made almost exclusively in the ovaries. They begin to flood the circulation when a girl starts to menstruate. Women who for one reason or another do not menstruate are particularly liable to osteoporosis. Obviously this will occur most often in women who naturally lose their menstrual periods after the menopause, but it also happens to women whose ovaries do not work properly or whose ovaries have had to be removed because of disease. Conversely women who in their lifetime have had more oestrogens in their circulation will be less liable to osteoporosis; this means women who start menstruating early, who stop late, who have had several children or who have used the contraceptive pills (which contain oestrogens).

Corticosteroids

The adrenal glands, which sit on top of the kidneys, make corticosteroid hormones that are essential to life. Without them the body cannot respond to the stresses of infection and trauma. When given as treatment these hormones reduce inflammation. Since their discovery and manufacture they have been used, sometimes in large amounts, to treat many diseases. An excess of these hormones, either in the illness called Cushing's syndrome or due to their excessive use as drugs, leads to a gain in weight, a rounded face, an increase in blood pressure, a thin and easily bruised skin and, most

13

relevantly, to bones becoming osteoporotic and brittle.

Other hormones
The adrenal glands also produce the building blocks that make up the sex hormones; these can be turned into active sex hormones in body fat. In women this becomes an important source of sex hormones after the menopause, when the ovaries have lost their activity.

The thyroid gland also makes a hormone called thyroxin, which has the effect of speeding up all body processes. Too much thyroxin causes loss of weight, palpitations, weakness, nervousness and a feeling of being inappropriately warm. Such people also lose bone faster than they make it and if untreated for long enough they become osteoporotic and their bones brittle.

Local hormones
The majority of other messengers or hormones that act on bone are made locally in or near bone. Some stimulate the formation, others the loss of bone. This is an area of great interest to researchers at present; if we can understand the fine tuning of bone growth then we may be able to influence it to prevent or reduce bone loss.

3

CAUSES OF OSTEOPOROSIS

BONE FRACTURE THRESHOLD

Any bone will break if the injury is severe enough. However in the elderly, broken bones often result from relatively slight injuries; the brittleness of their bones is greater, as is their chance of falling and causing themselves injury.

The concept of a 'fracture threshold' has therefore developed. This means that a bone has become so weak that it cannot be expected to stand up to the ordinary trivial accidents of daily life. Because women have smaller skeletons than men to start with, and because they lose calcium more rapidly as they get older, they arrive at this 'fracture threshold' much earlier than do men. Once they have crossed the 'fracture threshold' a broken bone is increasingly likely.

Which bones are most vulnerable at any age depends on the amount of bone mass lost from them. This in turn depends on the proportions of cortical (tubular) and trabecular (mesh-work) bone, as these show different rates of loss with age. Trabecular bone is more rapidly lost in women following the menopause, but there is also a slow but constant loss of cortical bone in both men and women from mid-life. As the bone is lost, the cortex thins and trabeculae are lost, which results in the increased fragility of the bone.

From this it would appear that we will all inevitably get osteoporosis if we live long enough. And to a certain extent that is true. We all lose bone with ageing, but only some of us will suffer the consequences. Although one in four women will sustain a fracture in later life, three out of four will not. So what

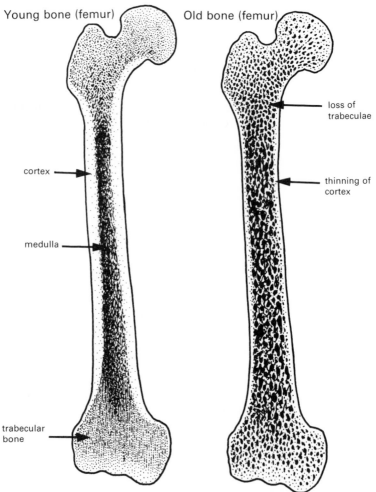

Young bone (femur)

Old bone (femur)

loss of
trabeculae

cortex

thinning of
cortex

medulla

trabecular
bone

Changes in the bone due to osteoporosis

is it which causes us all to lose bone as we age? Why do some of
us have insufficient bone when elderly? And what causes only
some of us to suffer the consequences – a broken bone? These
are questions which need to be looked into in detail.

FACTORS INVOLVED IN OSTEOPOROSIS

The amount of bone in the skeleton increases from conception
to about age 30, and then declines. The chance of suffering a

fracture of the hip, wrist and spine increases with age from mid-life. This coincidence of the loss of bone and increase in fractures strongly suggests that one leads to the other. However not everyone with osteoporotic bones breaks them. An injury such as a fall has to occur first and factors that affect the occurrence and severity of falls will also determine who does or doesn't break a bone. We therefore have to consider not only the causes of osteoporotic bones when we are old but also the causes of falls.

Another important consideration is not simply that the whole skeleton becomes weaker but that some bones are affected more than others. We talk of the skeleton as being a single entity, but in fact the bones in the skeleton react differently in different parts, and loss of bone strength is not universal and equal in all bones. For example, things would obviously be different if bone was lost from the flat bones of the skull rather than from the bones in the spine; the former is seldom exposed to much force but the spine is continually taking the weight of the body and will be much more likely to crush if weakened.

So, firstly, what determines how much bone you have when you are 70 years of age? This is the result of how much bone you developed at your peak at 35 years of age (your 'peak bone mass'), at what age you began losing bone and how fast you have been losing bone since then. Of these three, though, peak bone mass appears to be the most important.

PEAK BONE MASS

Peak bone mass is determined by genetics, nutrition, exercise in youth and sex hormones.

Genetics

Identical twins come from a single egg and therefore share the same inherited characteristics, while non-identical twins come from different eggs and therefore have different inherited characteristics. From studies made on the skeletons of identical and non-identical twins it has been noted that identical twins have skeletons with greater similarities than non-identical twins.

This is one demonstration of the fact that the characteristics of your skeleton are inherited from your parents; parents with thick or heavy bones generally have children who will grow up to have thick or heavy bones.

Diet

Good general nutrition is important for good health. In particular, adequate calcium and vitamin D during growth is important for the normal development of the skeleton. Curiously, though, malnourished adults in the third world do not suffer much from osteoporosis – they probably become more efficient at absorbing calcium from their limited diets.

Lack of vitamin D leads to weak bones, and lifelong diets deficient in calcium result in less bone and more fractures. This was nicely shown by studying two towns in Yugoslavia that were similar apart from their calcium intakes; in one town there was a high calcium intake and in the other a low one. The women in the calcium-rich district had denser bones and suffered fewer hip fractures than their compatriots in the low-calcium district.

Exercise

Exercise is also important – using a limb stimulates the growth of bone in it. For example, the right arms of right-handed professional tennis players have thicker bones than their left arms, when for most of us they would be about equal. Similarly, the bones which support the toes in ballet dancers become very much thicker when they are doing a lot of dancing which includes going up on their toes.

Conversely adults or children who are put into bed for a long time rapidly lose calcium from their bones. A similar thing happens to astronauts while they are weightless in space. Paralysis of a limb – after a stroke, poliomyelitis or multiple sclerosis – will also result in loss of calcium from the bones of that limb.

People with severe arthritis also lose bone strength because they cannot walk around normally. In addition, they may be treated with cortisone (corticosteroid)-like drugs which worsen this. Furthermore the inflammation of the joints results in a loss of calcium from the bone near the joint – local osteoporosis. It will be no surprise, therefore, to learn that some people with arthritis are more troubled by osteoporosis than by their joints.

Exercise is therefore good for bones, but there is one reservation. Competitive women athletes and ballet dancers sometimes train and diet so hard that they stop menstruating. They then actually have less bone than their menstruating colleagues. This shows that female sex hormones are more important in preserving bone than is exercise.

Sex hormones

The exposure of women to their female sex hormones is another factor determining the amount of bone they have at mid-life. Starting menstrual periods early, finishing late, using the contraceptive pill, having more pregnancies are all factors that favour more bone mass at mid-life. The rapid and predictable loss of bone after the removal of the ovaries also demonstrates the importance of these hormones.

ONSET OF BONE LOSS

What determines the age at which men begin to lose bone is unclear, but in women it is the menopause. The earlier the menopause, the sooner this loss of bone starts and the sooner the amount of bone in the skeleton will fall below the fracture threshold.

RATE OF BONE LOSS

Some people lose bone faster than others. Lack of calcium may be important in some and lack of exercise contributes in others, but where the cutoff lies between the idle and the fit in maintaining the strength of the skeleton is not established. In animals quite a small amount of vigorous daily exercise, roughly equivalent to running up and down stairs, is sufficient to prevent osteoporosis, while in post-menopausal women, three hours of aerobics a week has been shown to be effective.

Lack of female sex hormones also affects the rate of loss; it is fastest in those who have had their ovaries removed surgically because they have an almost total loss of female sex hormones. However obesity is protective as hormones from the adrenal glands can be made into female sex hormones by body fat. This is one case where being slim is not of benefit but is actually a risk factor for developing osteoporosis.

A lot of protein, caffeine and alcohol in the diet, as well as cigarette smoking, are all factors which speed up the loss of bone from the skeleton. And some specific conditions may also result in bone loss, for example: rheumatoid arthritis; treatment with corticosteroids; overactivity of the thyroid gland (hyperthyroidism, thyrotoxicosis); causes of immobility (stroke, polio, multiple sclerosis); liver diseases and chronic lung diseases.

4

OSTEOPOROSIS – WHO IS AT RISK?

This is the key question. In theory we are all at risk to some extent and the longer we live, the greater the risk. But obviously the risk is much more for some people than others, because in practice only one in four women is going to develop an osteoporosis fracture and only one in 40 men will do so.

Most osteoporosis can be prevented, but to do this we need to be able to pick out who is most likely to get it. And because prevention probably has to start many years beforehand if it is to be successful, we need in most instances to be thinking 10 to 20 years ahead. Doctors, like everyone else, have some difficulty in seeing into the future, and the further into the future that one is looking, the more difficult it becomes.

So is it impossible to prevent osteoporosis? The answer is, no. We can already recognise some situations where osteoporosis is inevitable and others where the risk is high. So people in these risk groups can be given preventive treatment. Then there are others where the risk factors seem to be pointing that way; here the task is to keep an eye on them, perhaps with repeated measurements to see if their bones are losing mineral abnormally fast – something which one cannot assess on a single measurement. Then there are people who show no signs of getting osteoporosis, or who may even have what are called 'negative risk factors', that is, conditions in which osteoporosis is unlikely.

Put this way, the task of selecting who to treat, who to watch and who to reassure and not see again becomes more simple.

WHEN OSTEOPOROSIS IS INEVITABLE

Osteoporosis can be predicted with considerable certainty in certain diseases and following certain treatments. In some of these it is associated with osteomalacia, a different bone disease caused by the failure of action of vitamin D, but this is separately treatable (see Chapter 10).

Premature menopause – the change of life

The average age of the menopause (when the periods stop) in women is 52, but that average covers quite a wide normal range – from about 45 to 60 years.

The earlier the menopause, however, the greater the risk of osteoporosis later. Some women lose their periods at 35, and others have to have their ovaries removed because of disease, such as endometriosis, ovarian cysts or ovarian cancer. For them, all the usual post-menopausal problems such as hot flushes, sweats and emotional instability are likely to come on quite severely, and most doctors would consider it almost unethical not to offer treatment with hormone replacement therapy. However what is not always realised is that this should be continued for many years, possibly until age 60 or more, if the almost inevitable osteoporosis is also to be avoided.

There are also a number of uncommon conditions in which the ovaries cease to work. One of the less rare ones is a condition in which one of the small glands, the pituitary, in the skull over-produces a hormone called prolactin. This is usually due to a tumour of the gland, called a prolactinoma. The normal function of this hormone is to switch on the production of breastmilk after a baby is born, but if the hormone is produced at the wrong time it suppresses the action of the ovaries. It can be a difficult problem to diagnose because, unless it is severe, it may not actually cause inappropriate milk production, even though it suppresses the ovaries. Today a simple blood test will give the answer. Then either the tumour is removed, or if it is small, supplementary ovarian hormones are given to overcome its effects.

Treatment with cortisone-like drugs

The adrenal gland produces small amounts of a hormone, hydrocortisone, which is essential to life. It was discovered how to make this synthetically, and tested in rheumatoid arthritis patients in 1948. These patients felt dramatically better because, given in large doses, hydrocortisone suppresses inflammation, including the painful inflammation of the joints which is characteristic of rheumatoid arthritis. Unfortunately there was a price to be paid, and part of that price was osteoporosis.

Today hydrocortisone and its close relative cortisone are rarely used. Instead, more convenient or more powerful derivatives are given; as a family of drugs they are known as corticosteroids or, sometimes, steroids.

The chief danger of osteoporosis arises when corticosteroids are given by mouth in large amounts for a long time. Corticosteroids are also well absorbed through the skin or when given by injection. Attempts are made by the manufacturers to limit the general absorption when only a local action is needed; for example, triamcinolone is often injected directly into painful swollen joints in arthritis but in a relatively slowly dissolving form, so that most of it stays where it is put. Even so, some is absorbed from the joint and can contribute to osteoporosis if too much is used, or too many joints are injected all at the same time.

Corticosteroid skin ointments are not without their problems; there are a large number of these ointments, some weak,

Corticosteroids in use today

Corticosteroid	Approximate equivalent dose in milligrams
Hydrocortisone	25
Cortisone	25
Prednisolone	5.0
Prednisone	5.0
Methylprednisolone	4.0
Triamcinolone	4.0
Betamethasone	0.5
Dexamethasone	0.5

some strong, and they have a large variety of trade names which may not make it obvious that they contain corticosteroids. The risk is greatest in such troublesome diseases as psoriasis, chronic eczema and dermatitis, where they are used over large areas of the skin.

There is one corticosteroid, called deflazacort, which in experimental conditions is less likely to cause osteoporosis. However, at the time of writing it is not generally available, and more experience of it is needed before we know how advantageous it is.

Whether or not corticosteroid treatment leads to osteoporosis depends on three things – the dose, the duration of treatment and the individual. Some individuals seem to be more resistant than others, perhaps because they have a high bone stock. Taking prednisolone as an example, merely because it is the most commonly used, a dose of 10 mg a day continued for three years will almost certainly cause significant osteoporosis, with the risk being greater in women than men. The same would be true of, say, 20 mg a day continued for one year or 7.5 mg a day for five years.

The risk of getting osteoporosis is not necessarily a reason for abandoning the use of corticosteroids. They may be literally life saving or eyesight saving, or they may make life tolerable to people suffering from severe asthma, eczema, or certain blood diseases. But it is a reason for remembering (and unfortunately too many doctors forget) that if they have to be given regularly over a long period of time, other things should be done to reduce the risk of osteoporosis; these include the possibilities of hormone replacement treatment in women, and the use of calcium and fluoride supplements, and will be discussed later.

Chronic liver diseases
Osteoporosis is inevitable in *primary biliary cirrhosis, chronic active hepatitis* and *haemochromatosis*. These are long words and need explaining. Luckily these liver diseases are all rare.

In **primary biliary cirrhosis** the body seems to mount an immune reaction to the bile ducts within the liver – it treats them as though they did not belong there, just as it might treat invading micro-organisms. The subsequent inflammation around the bile ducts leads to scarring of the whole liver. Eventually the bile ducts become blocked and jaundice

24

develops because the bile, which contains a yellow pigment, cannot get out into the gut. But long before this stage the action of the liver cells is interfered with.

Everything we eat, once it has been digested and absorbed through the wall of the intestine, has to pass through the liver, where it is processed so that nothing toxic gets into the main bloodstream. If the liver is not working, the proportion of calcium in the food which is absorbed falls. The liver is also responsible for converting vitamin D, either from our food or made by the action of sunlight on the skin, into its final very active state. This, too, fails in primary biliary cirrhosis, as the scarring process gets worse.

At present we cannot cure primary biliary cirrhosis. Luckily, though, it is only very slowly progressive in most people who have it, and there is quite a large proportion of sufferers who are quite unaware that they even have the problem – it may only be picked up in certain routine blood tests done for other reasons. Primary biliary cirrhosis mainly affects older women.

Chronic active hepatitis is a similar condition, but rather more serious. It affects younger people, and the target which the immune system is attacking is the liver cells themselves. In not all cases, however, is it severe, and it can be treated with corticosteroids, although, of course, these further increase the likelihood of osteoporosis.

Although **haemochromatosis** is a different liver disease, the results as far as the liver is concerned are much the same. It is the result of a failure to deal with iron in the body. Iron in the diet, in trace amounts, is essential for making healthy red blood cells; people who are deficient in iron become anaemic and pale. But most of us get more iron in our diet than we need, and we simply absorb what is necessary from the food we eat. In haemochromatosis, which mainly affects older men, too much iron is absorbed and, as it cannot easily be got rid of, it is 'dumped' in liver cells and in other parts of the body, including the skin, which literally becomes 'rusty'.

In all these conditions osteoporosis and some degree of osteomalacia is inevitable. The osteomalacia can be easily treated by giving small amounts of the active principle of vitamin D, which can now be made synthetically, while the osteoporosis can be reduced by increasing the calcium intake.

Malabsorption states

Osteoporosis becomes almost inevitable if the constituents of the diet needed to build healthy bones are not available or, if available, cannot be absorbed because of diseases which affect the digestion of food or alter the lining of the gut.

Of course, the most obvious such problem will be simple starvation. This is what happens to young women (and occasionally young men) who get the condition known as anorexia nervosa, the 'slimmer's disease'; for psychological reasons, they develop an aversion to food. Either they do not eat it, or if they do eat it they immediately vomit. As a result they become thinner and thinner, and eventually lose all their body fat. Surprisingly they may tell you they feel well, and may remain quite strong for weeks, until they eventually become very ill. Women with anorexia nervosa usually lose their periods because, as a result of the starvation, the ovaries no longer work to produce female sex hormones.

Osteoporosis is inevitable in these people. If they can be persuaded to eat normally, their periods will return, and their bones will recover to some extent – this has been shown by studies of their bone density. But a minority get into a state when they continue to eat only a minimum diet and, although they survive, their periods do not return. They are then in much the same situation as women who have a premature menopause.

In other people the problem is not that they refuse to eat, but that what they eat is not properly absorbed. Commonest are those people who have had to have a gastrectomy – removal of part or all of the stomach – usually because of serious ulceration of the stomach or duodenum. One can survive without a stomach but food is not properly digested and the lining of the intestine becomes damaged and does not absorb as well as it should.

There are many causes of malabsorption, such as sensitivity to gluten, the protein found in wheat flour, or loss of the enzymes called disaccharidases which allow us to digest and absorb ordinary sugar or milk sugar. Many of these problems are treatable if correctly diagnosed. Some are not, however, and if they persist long enough calcium will not be absorbed properly, nor will vitamin D, and osteoporosis and osteomalacia may result.

WHEN OSTEOPOROSIS IS UNLIKELY

Men
Very few men get osteoporosis – 39 out of 40 men will not experience an osteoporosis-related fracture, of those that do get it, in more than half the cases it is the result of some other condition or treatment such as corticosteroids. So it is not worth setting up a general screening process for men.

Women
There is one category of women who, although not immune, is very unlikely to show osteoporosis. Not that they get off Scot-free – they are those women who develop primary osteoarthritis. They are in fact 'bone formers', not 'bone removers'. They develop bony knobs, called osteophytes, around their joints, usually in response to excessive wear in the joints. Their hands show characteristic changes, with little knobs (called Heberden's nodes, after the 18th-century physician who first called attention to them). Women with primary osteoarthritis do get hip problems, caused by arthritis of the hip rather than a fracture of the hip. Since both these hip

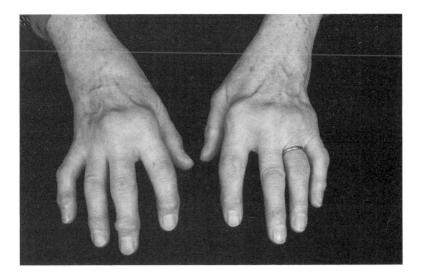

Osteoarthritis of the hands. The bony swollen joints of the fingers are caused by osteoarthritis and are known as Herberden's nodes. Women with this type of osteoarthritis are not likely to develop osteoporosis.

conditions are often treated by the same operation – total hip-joint replacement – it has been possible to study the hip joints in both osteoporosis and in osteoarthritis. And in general they are strikingly different. In osteoporosis the bone is soft, but the joint itself is intact, and there are no bony knobs around the edge of the joint. Exactly the opposite happens in osteoarthritis; the joint is misshapen, the natural self-lubricating cartilage has disappeared, there is a proliferation of new bone around the edges of the joint, and the bone itself is extremely hard. Like everything else in medicine, this tale – that if you have osteoarthritis you will not get osteoporosis – is not 100 per cent reliable, although nearly so.

Another, and much larger, group of women unlikely to get osteoporosis as they get older is women who in their lives have had a larger than usual experience of circulating sex hormones. Let us explain. This does not mean they have been more 'sexy' in the conventional sense of the word, but it does mean they probably started having their periods early, perhaps before age 13, and finished them late, perhaps after 55. In between they have had, and probably breastfed, several children. They have never been heavy smokers (smoking interferes with the action of female sex hormones, and even 'passive smokers', women who live in households where others smoke, lose their periods earlier than do non-smokers). They have had no serious debilitating illness – such as asthma or rheumatoid arthritis, and when they were not busy having a family they will have been on the contraceptive pill – which contains female hormones. On the whole they will have been somewhat overweight. Plump, jolly and fertile might be a general description of the women unlikely to develop osteoporosis. Other plus values might be that they have been keen on exercise, especially when younger, and they were well fed as children, with plenty of milk, a taste for which they carried into adult life.

To this general recipe for a woman to avoid osteoporosis, doctors can bring rather more sophisticated tests of bone density. If a woman arrives at the menopause with strong dense bones, she is unlikely to lose bone mineral in her post-menopausal life to the extent that her bones will fail in her 60s and beyond. Such machines for measuring bone density are as yet not very common in hospitals in Great Britain, nor are they 100 per cent accurate. But technology advances, and new generations of bone densitometers, as they are called, will soon be available and will be both more accurate and less expensive.

WHEN OSTEOPOROSIS IS POSSIBLE

Between the relatively few people for whom osteoporosis is almost inevitable unless prevented, and the relatively large number of people for whom osteoporosis is very unlikely, come the rest. By excluding these two groups it is possible to reduce the number of women 'at risk' to perhaps one in three – still not enough of a reduction to allow us to treat all of them in the hope of preventing it in the minority, but still an advance.

The doctor's strategy is therefore to review such women at, say, yearly intervals and pick out those who do not only have a number of risk factors – such as late onset of periods, early menopause, history of anorexia, heavy smoking, etc. – but who also have relatively less bone on bone-density measurements. The doctor will then have a base to work from. And if after a year the women is a 'fast bone loser' as judged by the bone densitometer, then she is clearly at risk.

From the risk factors we have discussed that increase the chances of osteoporosis and bone fracture, you can construct your own risk-factor profile. We do not know exactly the risk carried by each of these factors, but we have estimated this. Most consider the premature loss of female sex hormones to be the most important factor, while lack of calcium and of physical activity probably rate similarly. Being too thin also scores another risk factor. In this way we can try and work out a score sheet. We cannot yet pick out everybody who will become osteoporotic, but at least it is an attempt to give you and your doctor some guidance as to whether to seek preventive treatment before suffering a fracture.

This is the time to recognise the problem, before it has developed, as we can prevent osteoporosis with hormone replacement therapy, helped by calcium supplementation. Unfortunately as yet we have no cure for it once it is firmly established.

Osteoporosis risk profile for women

The bold lines indicate the relative importance – big risk factors have longer lines than small risk factors. See what applies to you.

Category of risk	Possible risk	Small risk	Medium risk	Definite risk
Personal risk factor				
Mother or grandmother had osteoporosis	▬			
Started periods after age 15	▬▬▬	▬		
Finished periods before age 45	▬▬▬	▬▬	▬	
Never pregnant	▬▬▬	▬		
One pregnancy only	▬▬▬	▬		
Never on the 'contraceptive pill'	▬▬▬	▬		
Cigarette smoker (10 or more a day)	▬▬▬	▬▬		
Underweight for height	▬▬▬	▬		
Not fond of games or exercise when child	▬▬▬	▬		
Not fond of games or exercise when adult	▬▬▬	▬		
Diet				
Milk generally avoided – less than ½ pint a day	▬▬▬	▬▬	▬	
Cheese disliked	▬▬▬	▬▬	▬	
Other dairy products (yoghurt, ice cream) avoided	▬▬▬	▬		
Eats lots of meat and fish	▬			
Takes extra roughage (fibre) in diet	▬			
Illnesses				
Anorexia when younger	▬▬▬	▬▬	▬▬	▬
Thyroid gland overactive in past	▬▬▬	▬▬	▬	
Treatment with thyroid hormones	▬▬▬	▬		
Treatment with corticosteroids				
as pills	▬▬▬	▬▬	▬▬	▬
as ointments	▬▬▬	▬▬	▬	
as inhalant	▬▬▬	▬▬	▬	
Teeth fell out or removed when young	▬			
Previous broken bones				
once	▬▬▬	▬▬	▬	
several times	▬▬▬	▬▬	▬▬	▬

There is a total of 24 different categories of risk and 4 levels of risk, giving 96 combinations. You will see that the bold lines run through a total of 60 such combinations. If you score more than 30 it puts you in the 'likely to get osteoporosis' group.

RISK FACTORS FOR A FALL

For a bone to break not only must it be weak but you also need to fall. So anything that increases the risk of falling also increases the risk of breaking a bone.

Most falls occur in the home. It is not just the uneven or icy pavement that one has to be careful of – the loose rug in the lounge is more dangerous, as are pet dogs or cats, and children's toys left lying about. In addition to this, problems such as forgetting to wear one's glasses, dizzy spells and blackouts may all cause a fall. Staying in a strange house can cause you to fall on unseen steps. Tablets to reduce blood pressure may make you feel unsteady when you first stand up – pausing for a few moments before moving will help. Sleeping pills may make you lose balance when you get up in the morning.

Our reflexes are slower when we get older and there is often less muscle and fat to cushion a fall on an already weakened bone, with the result that one is more likely to end up with a fracture.

Osteoporosis can therefore be largely escaped by maintaining strong bones and avoiding falls.

5

SYMPTOMS OF OSTEOPOROSIS

How do you know if you have the beginnings of osteoporosis? The answer is that you will not – not until your bones begin to give way. Osteoporotic bones do not hurt, but feel perfectly normal until they break or crush. Even an ordinary X-ray of a bone will not show osteoporosis until a third of the bone mineral in it has been lost. Occasionally osteoporosis is detected by X-rays carried out for another reason but most often it is diagnosed when it is too late – enough bone has been lost for it to have broken with a trivial fall.

Instead of putting your arm out and saving yourself, you are on the floor with a broken wrist. Instead of getting up after tripping over the carpet, you lie on the floor in pain with a broken hip. Instead of jumping off the bus and walking away, you suddenly get a severe pain in the back as a bone in the spine crushes. Or you gradually become aware that you are stooping and shrinking in height. Perhaps you were eye to eye with your husband; now he can look over the top of your head. These are all the features of established osteoporosis.

The important thing is that a fracture should be recognised as a symptom of osteoporosis, and treatment to prevent worsening of this should be considered. Unfortunately, as is discussed later, the treatments that we have for established osteoporosis are not yet perfect but much can be done to reduce the risk of further bone fracture. This is important, as once somebody has suffered one osteoporotic fracture, then they are at risk of others. Much can also be done to make life more comfortable for the sufferer.

TESTING FOR OSTEOPOROSIS

Can we detect osteoporosis before a bone breaks? We have already stated that ordinary X-rays are not very good at showing the loss of bone from the skeleton before one-third has gone, but there are now several other ways to measure the amount of bone in the skeleton.

Single and dual photon absorptiometers (also known as densitometers) are used to measure the amount of mineral in bone and its density. This, in most people, is a good measure of its strength. A source of radiation is placed on one side of the body or limb and a collector is put on the other. Some of the radiation will be absorbed and stopped by the calcium in the bone. What does not pass through gives a measurement of the amount of calcium. Single photon absorptiometry can measure the amount of bone in the forearm, and dual photon absorptiometry can measure the amount of bone in the hip or spine. New methods based on the absorption of X-rays (dual energy X-rays) give a quicker result. Computerised tomography (which is based on X-rays) can also be used for the spine.

These machines are unfortunately very expensive and there are not many in use in the United Kingdom; they are more commonly available in the United States. They can measure the quantity of bone and show if it is less than you would expect for the average person of the same age and sex. If it is low then treatment may be appropriate to prevent further loss. The machines can then be used to see how well the treatment is working. These machines do not give all the answers as they only measure the amount of bone and not its strength, but they are useful for picking out those people at most risk of fracture as well as those unlikely to fracture unless the injury is severe.,

A bone biopsy, when a small piece of bone is painlessly removed from the pelvis bone, is sometimes performed to see if the quantity of bone is normal, and there are also some blood and urine tests that can show if bone is being removed too rapidly or formed too slowly. These tests are all used to identify people with osteoporosis before they actually come to the doctor with a broken bone, and to monitor the response to treatments. Other tests are sometimes necessary to look for other causes of bone pain or weakness.

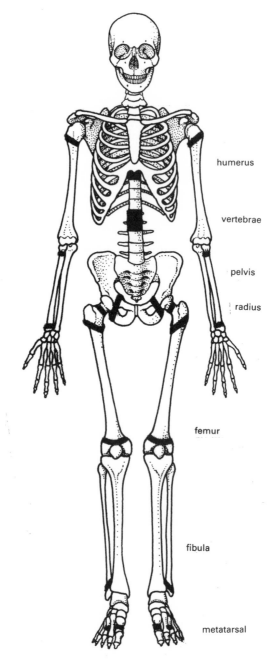

humerus

vertebrae

pelvis

radius

femur

fibula

metatarsal

Bones and points where fractures are most likely to occur

FRACTURES OF OSTEOPOROSIS

There are several places where bones commonly break in people over 50 years and which are considered to be related to osteoporosis.

- Wrist
- Neck of femur – the hip
- Neck of humerus – the shoulder
- Pelvis
- Vertebrae – the back bones

Wrist

If a young person falls heavily and puts out a hand to protect herself, the arm will usually break at the elbow. An elderly person, though, usually breaks the neck of the humerus (the bone in the upper arm, near the shoulder) or one of the bones of the lower arm, the radius, near the wrist (a Colles' fracture).

If the wrist is broken it will be painful and usually misshapen. At the hospital the doctors will line up the bones correctly, either under a local or general anaesthetic, and put the wrist in a plaster for four to six weeks. The pain usually settles after a few days but it will be difficult coping with everyday chores such as washing oneself, dressing and cooking with a plaster on one arm, and impossible if you live alone. Indeed, someone who lives alone may need to be looked after in hospital until the plaster is removed. Recovery from this fracture is usually complete.

Shoulder

Fracture of the shoulder at the top end of the humerus (the bone in the upper arm) is not so common and can be more troublesome. It is difficult to fix the bone fragments in their original position, so it is usually treated with a simple sling and left to heal in its new position. In the long term the shoulder will recover, but it will not be possible to use it as well as before; reaching for a high shelf, for example, or hanging washing on a line may become more difficult.

Hip

When the hip, or more accurately the proximal femur (top end of the thigh bone), breaks the problem is much more serious;

mobility and independence are often lost permanently.

The fracture may follow a fall, but some people actually feel their hip give way before they fall – their bone is simply so brittle it cannot take the stress of an ordinary step. The person is left lying on the floor waiting for their family or a friend to find them and get them to hospital. If they can drag themselves to a telephone or if they have a personal alarm system they will be able to get help earlier. The longer they are on the floor the more likely they are to get pneumonia; unfortunately many elderly people succumb to this.

Treatment for this sort of fracture used to be a long period of bed rest and traction, with the leg being pulled out, and many hip-fracture victims used to develop pneumonia or pressure sores in hospital. Nowadays, though, most people are operated on and either a new hip joint is fitted or the bones are pinned together with metal screws or nails. Following these operations patients are soon got out of bed and can be home within two weeks.

In hospital patients will receive physiotherapy to get them as mobile as possible. Before a patient with a hip fracture is sent home, an occupational therapist may visit the home to

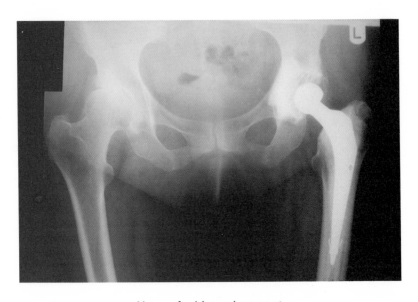

X-ray of a hip replacement

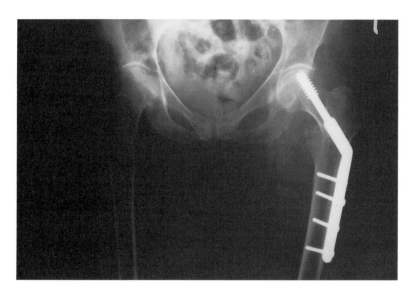
X-ray of a broken femur pinned together

ensure that the patient will be able to cope – that she can get upstairs to bed, on and off the toilet and in and out of the bath or shower. Aids may be provided to enable the patient to manage. If preparing meals is no longer possible then meals-on-wheels can be provided. If it is no longer possible to look after the home then a home help can be provided.

Although recovery from this fracture has improved enormously in recent years, many very elderly still do not get over all this and die within six months of the fracture; others do not get back to their previous level of independence and cannot cope alone at home any more. This is the fracture with the most long-term problems for the patient, the family and the medical and social services. This is the fracture that blocks hospital beds and costs the NHS many millions of pounds each year. Prevention of this fracture would have major benefits for all.

Pelvis

Less commonly the pelvis itself may break. This needs prolonged bed rest to heal and may result in loss of independence.

Feet

The bone in the middle of the foot – the metatarsals – can sometimes break without any obvious injury. This is known as a 'march fracture' because it sometimes occurs in young men in the army during a long march. Although initially painful, it heals without any long-term problems.

Ribs

A fall can also result in a cracked rib, although a loving hug or a cough may be sufficient to break an osteoporotic rib. Fractured ribs can be quite painful and there is a risk of developing pneumonia.

A cracked rib is treated by relieving the pain. There should be no long-term problems.

VERTEBRAE

Symptoms of osteoporosis of the spine

The spine consists of 24 blocks of bone, the vertebral bodies, separated from each other by rubbery cushions, the intervertebral discs. These cushion-like structures are under pressure, inflated not by air, as a rubber cushion might be, but by water semi-solidified into a kind of jelly and surrounded by a tough outer coat made of braided fibres.

Normally the strength of the vertebral bodies, the bones, keep these cushion-like discs flat. The first thing that happens in spinal osteoporosis is that the centre part of the intervertebral disc becomes more incompressible than the centre parts of the bones on each side of them. The discs then squash the bones which lie above and below them. On X-ray the bones now look more like fish vertebrae – they are hollowed out at each end or biconcave.

This process may or may not be painful. There are very few nerve-endings inside the bones and none inside the discs, although there are plenty on their surfaces. So in many cases these changes take place without the subject knowing or, if pain does occur, it may be accepted as just part of the aches and pains that most people get as they get older.

The next thing that happens is that a vertebral body begins to collapse. This happens at the front of the bone at first, so that it becomes wedged. The final stage occurs when the whole

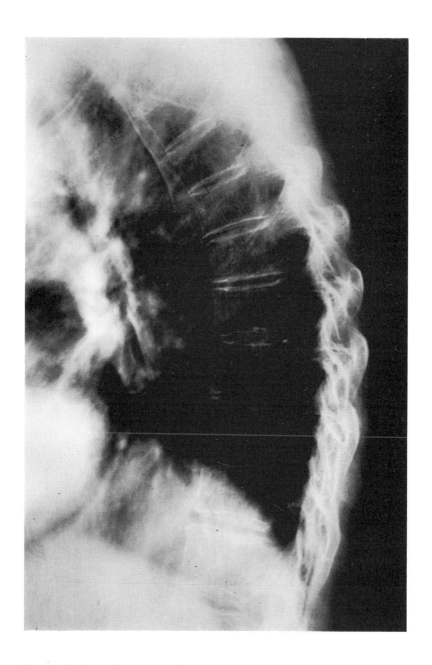

X-rays of the early stages of osteoporosis

a) Early osteoporosis with loss of bone

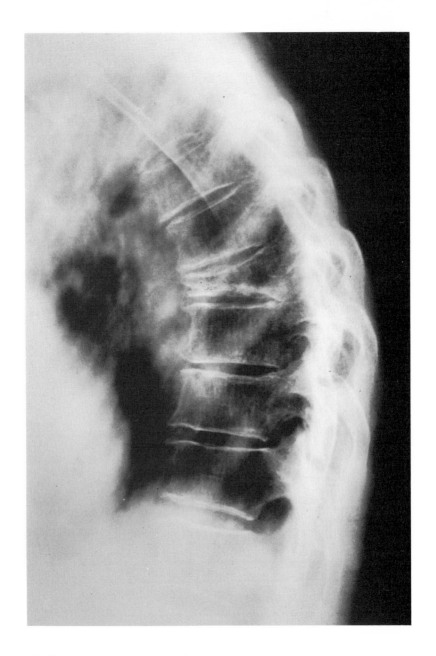

b) Progression to vertebral fracture

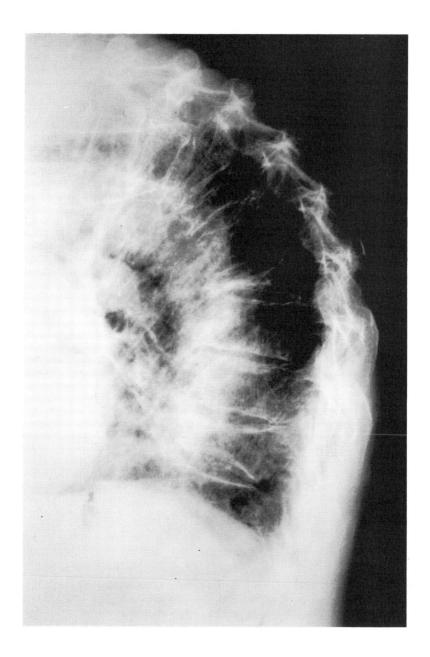

c) Further progression with several crushed wedge fractures

of the vertebral body becomes crushed and collapses. Of course, as there are 24 different vertebral bodies, the process may go on at different levels in the spine at different rates.

Acute vertebral-body crush-fracture syndrome

The symptoms of collapse of a vertebral body are characteristic but vary according to which bone is affected. Vertebral collapse may follow a fall or heavy lifting, or it may occur quite spontaneously. Usually the first symptom is severe pain. It occurs on stooping forwards, on trying to lift something heavy or sometimes when taking a rather steep step downwards and landing heavily on ones' feet. And the pain can be literally paralysing. The whole back goes into spasm and it is impossible to move, the face goes pale, and the sufferer often feels and may actually be sick.

Where the pain is felt depends on which part of the spine has had the crush fracture. The bones which are most often crushed are those at the bottom end of the thoracic spine (the chest region) and at the upper part of the lumbar spine (between the ribs and the top of the pelvis).

Surprisingly, pain is not felt only in the back but is usually felt in front as well. Sufferers describe it as 'a belt of pain' or 'vice-like', while doctors describe it as 'pain radiating around the body' or as 'referred pain'. This spread of pain from the back follows a pattern. For example, if it is the ninth thoracic (chest) vertebra the pain is felt along the bottom edge of the ribcage. If it is the eleventh thoracic vertebra it spreads around the abdomen at the level of the umbilicus (tummy button); this may be confusing and lead to the suspicion that something is wrong in the stomach. If it is the fifth thoracic vertebra, pain may spread across the chest and may be misdiagnosed as heart pain.

After a while the severe pain eases off. It may be in an hour or sometimes in a day or two, but it tends to strike again on movement, deep breathing, coughing or sneezing. Left to itself the pain gradually settles and usually clears up in anything from two to six weeks as the bone heals.

How the acute spinal crush fracture should be treated to help pain and minimise long-term damage is dealt with in Chapter 10.

Loss of height, rounding of the back

When a limb bone is fractured it heals back to the same shape

42

and length as it was before, provided it is set properly – there is no residual deformity. The opposite is true of spinal fractures. When they heal, the bone has changed shape and the person concerned is that much shorter. Moreover, it is mainly the front part of the bones of the spine which have crushed, so that a stoop will develop.

When several bones have crushed the loss of height and rounding of the back become prominent. Some women lose as much as 6 inches (15 cm) in height. When two or more vertebrae have crushed, this is known as 'established osteoporosis'.

It is a curious fact that a crush fracture is not inevitably painful. Some people with osteoporosis first go to their doctors having lost height and changed shape but with scarcely any pain. They have got to the point of established osteoporosis without the usual episodes of severe sudden pain.

ESTABLISHED SPINAL OSTEOPOROSIS

For someone with established spinal osteoporosis there are a number of other changes which may become more of a burden than the osteoporosis itself. They arise from the fact that, when the whole spine has shrunk, there is much less room in the chest and abdominal cavities than there used to be. Some of the consequences are obvious.

The chest
In the chest there is less room for the lungs to expand. It is impossible to take deep breaths, so sufferers find themselves easily short of breath after mild exertion. More seriously they may have difficulty in 'clearing their tubes' if they get a chest infection or pneumonia.

The abdomen
In the abdomen, the kidneys, liver and guts are just the same size as they used to be but there is now less room for them. So the abdomen protrudes forward.

Some sufferers first go to their doctors complaining they are getting fat. Others try to wear tight corsets to keep the bulge in. Of course this cannot be the solution; it only makes things worse. The body has 'concertina-ed' and often one can see

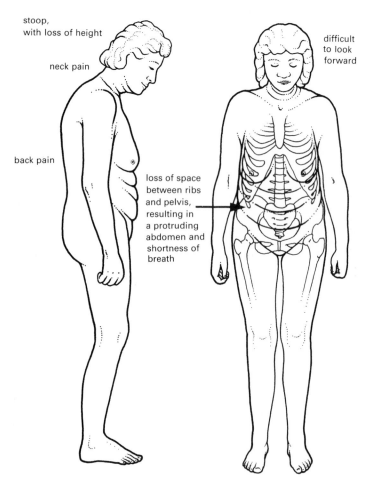

stoop,
with loss of height

neck pain

back pain

difficult
to look
forward

loss of space
between ribs
and pelvis,
resulting in
a protruding
abdomen and
shortness of
breath

pelvic floor weak with incontinence and coughing or sneezing

Problems in established osteoporosis

concertina-like folds in the skin around the abdomen when the trunk has got shorter.

With less room in the abdomen there is a tendency for the stomach to move upwards into the chest. This is called hiatus hernia, and is a common problem in osteoporosis. The acid stomach contents then make the lower end of the gullet sore and the unfortunate sufferer may get a chest pain or a feeling that food is sticking behind the breast bone.

At the other end of the abdomen is the pelvis, and increasing pressure here may mean difficulty in controlling the bladder – stress incontinence. This makes it necessary to go to the toilet frequently, and some women have to wear a pad because of leakage.

The ribs

Troubles do not end there. One test for spinal osteoporosis which doctors can do (and which you can do yourself) is to feel for the gaps between the bottom of the ribcage and the top of the pelvis at the side of the abdomen. Normally the gap is about three fingers wide, but in spinal osteoporosis the gap may be one finger or less.

In some women the ribs actually slide down inside the pelvis. If, as in many women, the pelvis is wide and the ribcage narrow, there will not be a collision, but in some people the ribs and pelvis collide painfully. Some have had lower ribs removed because of this.

The neck

As the spine shrinks, the back becomes more and more hunched and it becomes increasingly difficult to hold the head up when standing, either to see forward or, for that matter, to drink a glass of water standing up.

This problem in turn sets up strains in the neck muscles which become overactive and painful. Some women with established osteoporosis and a marked stoop get more pain from their necks than they do from their backs. The last stage of all comes when it becomes impossible to hold the head up without help. This is uncommon, though. At first the head can be pushed up with the hands and then held there by the muscles. Later the head comes to lie permanently chin on chest. A woman with this problem can only stand with difficulty and when doing so cannot see forward in order to look where she is going. The skin under the chin where it rubs against the chest, as well as the skin in the folds of the concertina creases around the abdomen, may become sore and infected.

The back

There may be chronic back pain. The new position of the spine

45

puts such strains on the joints and ligaments of the back that chronic pain occurs and may be very hard to treat.

To summarise, people with severe spinal osteoporosis will lose height, will often become easily breathless, will get symptoms of hiatus hernia, will have a bulging abdomen, may have difficulty controlling their bladder and may get pain from the ribs colliding with the pelvis or from strains in the neck muscles trying to hold the head up.

6

PREVENTION FROM CHILDHOOD TO MIDLIFE

The evidence strongly suggests that most osteoporosis can be prevented. Not everyone gets it – it is uncommon in men, for example. So it is not something which is an inevitable part of getting older.

However, the evidence also suggests that preventive measures, if they are going to be used, must be started in childhood. Children have to build strong bones that will last them a lifetime, and anything which interferes with bone building will make osteoporosis more likely later on, particularly in girls. We cannot pick out at this age those children who are most at risk and so these measures apply to all.

PREVENTION IN CHILDHOOD

With regular exercise, enough calcium and fluoride in the diet, and enough vitamin D from sunlight or food, children will make bones strong enough to last a lifetime.

Calcium

Children below the age of puberty have their own ways of ensuring the normal growth and development of the skeleton. For example, they have growth hormones that control the size of the skeleton, and they are much more efficient than adults at absorbing into their bloodstream the calcium which they receive in their diet.

Human breastmilk provides everything that is necessary for the nursing baby. Perhaps not surprisingly it is quite different in composition from cow's milk; compared to calves, babies grow slowly and do not have nice furry coats to keep them warm. So human breastmilk has about 50 per cent more sugar, to provide energy to keep the baby warm. However, it has less than half as much of the proteins which calves need for rapid growth and it also has only about a quarter as much calcium. It is when the baby is weaned and milk becomes only part of its diet, instead of all its diet, that cow's milk becomes particularly important as a source of calcium – no other food is so rich in calcium. The need for calcium is most important when children are growing rapidly between the ages of 9 and 14.

Calcium and milk

Calcium is so vital to babies before and after birth that a mother will provide it from her own body even if she herself is short of it. It is important, therefore, that she takes calcium supplements during pregnancy and breastfeeding or she will sacrifice her bones for the baby.

Once an infant is weaned, there is sometimes a change in its intestines. In such children, the gut can no longer digest lactose, the sugar which is present in milk, so the milk passes

United Kingdom recommended daily allowance (RDA) of calcium

Group	Age	RDA (milligrams)
Infants	0–1	600
Children	1–8	600
Adolescent	9–14	700
Young adults	15–17	500
Adult men	over 18	500
Adult women*	over 18	500
Pregnant women	—	1,200
Nursing mothers	—	1,200

*Adult women should, in the opinion of most authorities, be divided into those before the menopause, for whom an RDA of 500 mg is too low, and postmenopausal women, for whom the RDA should be above 1,500 mg.

How much calcium is there in foods?

Typical serving of	Amount	Calcium	% recommended daily allowance of 700 mg for adolescents
Whole milk	⅓ pint (190 ml)	230 mg	33
Semi-skimmed milk	⅓ pint (190 ml)	240 mg	34
Skimmed milk	⅓ pint (190 ml)	250 mg	36
Yoghurt	5 oz (150 g)	270 mg	38
Cheddar cheese	2 oz (60 g)	440 mg	63
Cottage cheese	4 oz (120 g)	60 mg	9
Dairy ice cream	6 oz (180 g)	68 mg	23
Tinned sardines	2 oz (60 g)	220 mg	31
Tinned salmon	2 oz (60 g)	46 mg	7
Prawns	2 oz (60 g)	75 mg	11
White bread	2 lge slices	60 mg	9
Wholemeal bread	2 lge slices	60 mg	9
Cabbage, broccoli, etc.	4 oz (120 g)	30–80 mg	4–11
Baked beans	4 oz (120 g)	45 mg	6
Red kidney beans	4 oz (120 g)	140 mg	20
Peanuts and other nuts	4 oz (120 g)	68 mg	10

Lean meat, chicken and fish, although excellent foods, are relatively poor sources of calcium.

right through the gut and may cause diarrhoea. Probably no more than 5 per cent of infants and children have this problem, but they soon make the connection that milk gives them colic and diarrhoea and they 'go off' milk. This means, of course, that they lose one of the richest food sources of calcium. Fortunately, if the problem is recognised, it is very easy to overcome it by adding an enzyme from yeast to the milk overnight in the refrigerator. This breaks down the milk sugar to other easily digested (and also sweeter) sugars. This is worth remembering when children who need milk refuse it.

Of course, the milk does not have to be whole milk. All the calcium is in the non-fat part of milk and none in the cream, so those who are worried about their children getting too fat or taking animal fats can use skimmed milk or low-fat yoghurts and cheeses. Children who don't like milk may often take it in the form of flavoured drinks or cooked as custards and milk puddings.

In Russia, after the revolution, there was an enormous amount of malnutrition. In order to get over this the authorities mounted a campaign to get everyone to eat ice cream made with milk. As a result the general level of nutrition improved, particularly the level of calcium, enabling children to build bigger and stronger bones. In Japan after the Second World War children on a low-calcium diet were given added milk. Similarly in Britain, when a third of a pint of milk was available free of charge to all schoolchildren, there was a striking increase in the rate of their growth and in their eventual height as adults.

Calcium and bread

When wholemeal flour is refined into white flour, most of the calcium is taken out. Studies in Newcastle upon Tyne showed clearly that less well-off children would get less than the minimum daily requirement of calcium in their diets if the government allowed millers to stop adding calcium to bread flour – something which had been compulsory for them in order to improve childrens' health and growth since wartime.

Today all white bread flour is fortified to bring it up to the level of wholemeal flour. Paradoxically, the calcium in white bread flour is more available for absorption than that in the original flour, and it contributes significantly to the needs of growing children in poorer families.

Exercise and bones

The importance of developing strong bones in childhood that will last a lifetime cannot be over-emphasised. The role of food had been mentioned – particularly its calcium content – but of equal if not greater importance is regular and reasonably vigorous exercise. This is recognised by everybody – schools, colleges, government – but in practice it too often doesn't happen.

It is the girls, who are most at risk of osteoporosis when they grow up, who are most likely to miss out. Pressures, such as swotting for exams, take up their time and stop them taking exercise. There are still 'Victorian' ideas around that it is not 'ladylike' for girls to run and play in competitive games. And on top of this there are some societies and religions which actively discourage girls from any form of exercise, including dancing, regarding it as slightly immoral. Finally expenditure on sport in schools is one of the first things to go if economies have to be made. Parents thus have an even greater responsibility to see that their children get regular exercise and activity. And this exercise should be outside in the sun if possible; calcium which is so essential for bones is not properly absorbed from food unless there is sufficient vitamin D present, and for most people up to 90 per cent of the vitamin D they need is made by the action of sunlight on their skin.

Exercise stimulates bones to grow and to remain strong in ways that are not yet fully understood. It seems that the living cells in bones have ways of measuring just how much force is being exerted on a bone – a lot of force, and they build stronger bones, too little and the bone cells become lazy and the bones weaken. Astronauts in space are weightless, without the force of gravity on them, and they rapidly lose calcium from their bones unless they perform a special exercise routine. People who get put to bed for any reason for a long time lose calcium. Conversely bones which are used strongly become even stronger – the right arm in professional tennis players or the foot bones in ballet dancers are examples. A child's limb which can't be used properly, perhaps because of previous infantile paralysis (poliomyelitis), has weak bones and fails to grow properly.

Fluoride and bones
Fluoride is an essential trace element, like iodine, copper, manganese or selenium. Only minute quantities of trace elements are needed, but without these minute quantities proper growth or even life itself is in danger. All trace elements therefore are very powerful and are poisonous if given in too great a quantity.

Young animals reared on diets which contain no fluoride get weak bones, bad teeth and they cannot grow properly. However, growth is restored if a trace of fluoride is added to their food. The amount of fluoride needed is exceedingly small; there is usually enough in the domestic water supply to satisfy the needs of growing children as most natural water contains a trace of fluoride – about one to two parts per million. When water comes partly from melted snow, as it does in mountainous districts or in northern countries, it may be deficient in fluoride.

In Britain, children's tooth-decay rate has fallen strikingly in areas where the drinking water has had fluoride added in trace amounts. This was made obvious by comparing Birmingham which has fluoridated water with nearby Wolverhampton, which has a similar water supply but without fluoride, where the decay rate remained high. In Finland, where the water has almost no fluoride in it, the women in one town developed twice as many osteoporosis-related hip fractures compared with women in another town where fluoride was added at one part per million.

Chemists sell, and doctors and dentists may prescribe, 1-mg-size tablets of sodium fluoride to help prevent dental decay in low-fluoride water supply districts. One tablet a day is all that is needed – containing about as much as would rest on the head of a pin. Not only will it help prevent tooth decay, it will also help build strong bones for children.

Vitamin D, the sunshine vitamin

Vitamin D is needed for calcium to be absorbed from the gut and for the normal formation of bone. Most of the vitamin D we need comes from the effect of the sun's ultraviolet light acting on building blocks of vitamin D present in the skin; the sunlight turns them into the active vitamin. So it is important to get out and about in the sun. Children who are always indoors or in cars are in some danger of being short of vitamin D because ultraviolet light will not go through ordinary window glass.

This vitamin is also found in foods such as margarine, which is fortified with vitamin D, in oily fish such as sardines, mackerel and herrings, and in fish-liver oils. But do not take too much. Vitamin D is one of the vitamins which are poisonous if used in excess, and tablets or capsules should not be needed in the young; 400 international units a day is all that is required.

CHILDHOOD TO MIDDLE LIFE

Bones stop growing in length at the end of childhood, about age 16–18 in girls and 18–20 in boys. However, they do not stop getting stronger. Bones are at their hardest and densest at the age of 35. Then they get less dense, very slowly at first until, in women, the time of the menopause, when the loss of bone density gets more rapid.

The ultimate strength of bones at age 35 and the rate at which bones get less strong after that age depend very much on the same three main things which were important in childhood – exercise, calcium, and traces of fluoride in the water supply. However, after puberty a new factor, the influence of the sex hormones, comes into play – androgens in boys, oestrogens in girls. These have an additional effect in promoting bone strength and indeed may override other influences.

Exercise

Sports and exercise will help them keep their bones strong, but how much exercise is needed? The evidence from experiments in adult animals suggests that surprisingly modest amounts will do. If sheep are unable to exercise they get osteoporosis, but even allowing them a brief walk around twice a day will prevent or minimise this. The human animal, on this count, would need to walk about 1½ miles (2½ km) a day or have a brisk run twice a day. This would probably maintain bones, although it wouldn't increase bone strength; for that, much more vigorous exercise is needed. Athletes and professional sportspeople commonly have stronger bones than more sedentary men and women.

For women the situation is more complicated. They are, of course, much more at risk of eventually getting osteoporosis, so exercise for them can also be recommended. But there is a limit. This is because female athletes, dancers and sportswomen may train themselves so hard and diet themselves so rigorously that they lose their menstrual periods, in which case, despite the intense exercise, they become osteoporotic. And an added complication is that they also lose almost all their body fat – and body fat is one of the tissues in the body which help produce female sex hormones.

Calcium

Although no longer growing in size, the skeleton becomes more dense from late teenage to midlife because calcium is still being deposited in the bones. Calcium remains important, therefore; it appears that a good intake of calcium throughout life leads to the maintenance of calcium levels in the bones and less chance of them breaking when older. During this time the actual amount of calcium needed in the diet is not as great as for the growing adolescent or the postmenopausal woman. Vitamin D is still necessary to facilitate the absorption of calcium, so keep getting enough (not excessive) sunshine on the skin. Vitamin D tablets or cod-liver oil should not be necessary if you go out of doors and occasionally eat fish.

Diet

We have already said that some body fat is of advantage when it comes to maintaining the strength of the skeleton. A woman who is overweight develops stronger bones, partly because of the extra weight that she has to carry around which requires both stronger bones and muscles. For example, a woman who weighs 15 stone (95 kg) when she ought to weigh 11 stone (70 kg) is carrying around with her the equivalent of half a bag of cement all the time! However, she keeps stronger bones, partly because of the extra fat she has – this you will remember, increases the amount of bone-protecting female sex hormones in the circulation (see page 19).

In contrast, people who are thin often have weaker bones. At the extreme there is a curious, partly psychological, condition which mainly affects young women – anorexia nervosa, the slimmers' disease. The young woman who has this may claim a distaste or revulsion for all food, yet (at first) remains apparently strong and active; gradually, though, she gets thinner and thinner and eventually loses her normal sex hormones and menstrual periods. Her bones are particularly liable to osteoporosis. Moreover when she gets better, as most do, the loss of calcium from her bones is only partly restored.

Sex hormones

As we have seen (page 13), the circulating sex hormones are important for the maintenance of healthy strong bones, so the length of time a woman has these hormones circulating around her body is therefore significant. The younger the age at which the menstrual period begins, the more pregnancies she has, and the use of the contraceptive pill all will protect a woman to some extent against getting osteoporosis in later life.

Smoking

Women are also disadvantaged when it comes to smoking. Cigarette smoking interferes with the production of female sex hormones. Furthermore, women smokers have an earlier menopause (and are therefore more inclined to get osteoporosis) than do women non-smokers – women smokers may lose as much as 5 years of premenopausal life. Even women non-smokers who live in households where there are heavy smokers are disadvantaged as they also get an earlier menopause.

7

PREVENTION AFTER THE MIDLIFE

The skeleton reaches its peak strength at midlife. From that time on it begins to lose bone mineral in both men and women. For women there is then a five to ten year period of rapid loss, starting about the time of the menopause. Since women have less bone than men to begin with and also have this phase of more rapid loss, they end up with much weaker bones than do men when they are elderly and they are therefore more likely to break their bones. However research has shown that a lot of this bone weakening can be prevented.

THE MENOPAUSE

The word menopause means, literally, the last menstrual period. However, this is not exactly the same thing as failure of the ovaries to produce sufficient sex hormones.

What happens is this. At birth a baby girl has a large number of potential eggs in her ovaries. At the time of puberty the pituitary gland in the brain starts up a monthly cycle of activity. It produces two hormones, a follicle stimulating hormone (FSH) and a luteinising hormone (LH). These do not produce their effects directly, but act on the ovaries, causing the eggs to grow and, in turn, the ovary to produce the two female sex hormones, oestrogen and progesterone.

The egg grows in the ovary inside a nest of other cells, called the follicle, and it is these follicle cells that first produce oestrogen. In fact there are a number of these natural oestrogens, but the most important is called oestradiol. At about halfway between menstrual periods the ripe egg leaves

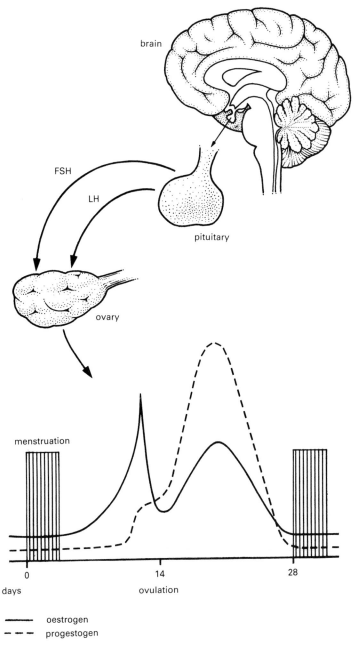

Changes in hormone level during the menstrual cycle

57

the ovary (ovulation) and begins to travel down towards the womb, ready to be fertilised. The follicle it has left behind does not disappear, but goes a yellow colour and, under the influence of LH, it secretes the sex hormone progesterone the function of which is to help build up the lining of the womb ready to receive the fertilised egg. An egg which is fertilised then attaches itself to the lining of the womb and sends a message to the ovary via the pituitary which says 'Keep making the progesterone'.

But if the egg is not fertilised, no message is sent to the pituitary and the stocks of progesterone are allowed to run down. The lining of the womb is then shed, along with the unfertilised egg – this is menstruation, a woman's period. The pituitary hormones then begin to stimulate another egg to ripen and to build up the lining of the womb again, and the whole process is repeated. This is the menstrual cycle.

If fertilisation occurs then the 'clock' of the pituitary is switched off, no further eggs are allowed to ripen and the fertilised egg stays in the womb as the baby grows. After the birth of the baby, the pituitary clock starts again and menstrual periods recur, although often this is not until breastfeeding (lactation) has finished.

This process goes on until about the age of 50, when the stock of eggs is nearly used up. Instead of ripening completely, the remaining eggs do so to a limited extent. The production of female sex hormones then dwindles. This reduction in circulating sex hormones is noticed by the pituitary which tries even harder, producing large amounts of the pituitary hormone FSH which normally drives the ovary to ripen more eggs – eggs that are no longer there. Doctors estimate when the menopause is likely to occur by measuring the amount of this pituitary hormone in the blood – the level of FSH rises before the menstrual periods cease. The physiological menopause is thus a gradual process and not a sudden one as the cessation of periods might imply; things are running down before the last menstrual period.

The various effects of the menopause are thought to be due to this overproduction of pituitary FSH and underproduction of female sex hormones.

For a fuller discussion of the menopause and how to cope with it see a companion book in this series, *The Menopause – Coping With The Change* by Dr Jean Coope.

PROBLEMS OF THE MENOPAUSE

The effects of the menopause on a woman can be divided under four headings:

- Effects on the circulation.
- Psychological effects.
- Effects on the pelvic organs – the sex organs and bladder.
- General loss of tissues (atrophy) – and this includes loss of bone leading to osteoporosis.

Effects on the circulation
The most common sign of the menopause are the hot flushes, which occur in up to 75 per cent of women. They may start before the last period and in some women they continue for five years or more after menstruation stops. Sometimes they are accompanied by sweating on the forehead and face. Sometimes also there are night sweats and waking up drenched. Some women get headaches and episodes of dizziness and fainting. These symptoms are alleviated by hormone replacement therapy.

Psychological effects
There are psychological changes at about the time of the menopause – depression, sleeplessness, irritability, mood swings from depression to over-activity – afflict some. A survey showed that nearly one in every two women who goes to her doctor about this time gets put on tranquillisers or similar drugs and some women subsequently get 'hooked' on them for life; many doctors still do not recognise that these symptoms are due to lack of oestrogens, not lack of tranquillisers. Other women notice a loss of concentration and a loss of desire for sexual activity.

Effects on pelvic organs
The vagina and uterus become smaller and the lining of the vagina becomes thin and dry. The natural lubrication decreases and the vagina becomes subject to infection fairly easily. Dryness may cause pain on making love. There is also some loss of pubic hair. The strength of the pelvic muscles becomes less. This means that some women lose control of the bladder when coughing and sneezing, a problem known as stress

incontinence. Sometimes there is prolapse of the uterus. All these changes can be reversed by hormone replacement therapy.

General atrophy

Thinning of the skin is easily confirmed by picking up a fold of skin on the back of the hand. The skin loses its elasticity because of loss of tissues and changes in the collagen fibres of the skin. There are also problems with the hair – a tendency to lose scalp hair and to develop a little moustache hair.

Women after the menopause have the same risk of atherosclerosis (hardening of the arteries) and coronary artery disease as do men, whereas before menopause they are less at risk. Women are more likely to suffer myocardial infarcts (heart attacks) after the menopause. This risk is also reduced with hormone replacement therapy.

THE MENOPAUSE AND THE SKELETON

The female sex hormones play an important part both in the development of the skeleton in women and in maintaining its strength. As we have seen, late onset of puberty and early onset of the menopause decrease the amount of bone in the mature skeleton. Bone mass is better maintained in women who have had a number of children and in women who have regularly taken oral contraceptives.

It was in the late 1930s that the idea was first proposed that osteoporosis follows loss of ovarian function. This was later proved in women who had their ovaries removed because of disease or tumour; this sudden loss of a woman's ovarian supply of sex hormones was shown to be followed by a rapid decrease in the density of the bones and an increase in the risk of osteoporotic fractures. It was also shown that this could be prevented by replacing the lost hormones. Nowadays no woman should have her ovaries removed before the time of natural menopause without being offered hormone replacement therapy.

HORMONE REPLACEMENT THERAPY AND THE SKELETON

Some of the best studies of hormone replacement therapy have been done on a group of women in Glasgow who have been followed since the late 1960s. They were women who had had their ovaries removed for various medical reasons. In those days it was not certain whether or not they should be given female hormone supplements, so some of them were given hormone replacement therapy (HRT) and some of them were not. Those not given HRT lost bone, but those treated with hormone replacement did not. And not only did the latter group keep better bones; they had fewer fractures.

Women have also been studied during and shortly after their natural menopause, and again results are quite clear. The bone loss which would have occurred is prevented by hormone replacement therapy. Once treatment is stopped bone begins to be lost again, but only at the rate it would have been before treatment, so that there is a permanent gain of the bone saved during the time the woman is on HRT.

An even more striking result came from a study of women in a town in the United States called Framingham. Framingham is famous in medicine because the medical history of the people who live there is known in great detail. All the women who fractured their hips in Framingham were followed up. It was shown that there were many more fractures in those who had not been on HRT than in those who had; any woman who had ever been on HRT had her risk of hip fracture reduced by one-third. If she was still taking HRT within two years of the follow-up the risk was reduced further, by two-thirds. And this was with 'old fashioned' techniques of HRT.

It is studies like this which give us confidence in saying that at least two out of every three hip fractures in older women are preventable. And that is a conservative estimate. Of all the treatments for osteoporosis, the benefits of hormone replacement therapy are the most certain.

Other benefits of HRT

Many elderly women die following an osteoporosis-related fracture of the hip – as many as one in four in some parts of the UK. HRT, by preventing osteoporosis, reduces the risk of such deaths.

It is also clear that HRT with oestrogen alone reduces the risk of ischaemic heart disease (heart attacks, coronary thrombosis) which is one of the major killers of women.

WHAT ARE THE PROBLEMS OF HRT?

There are very few problems with HRT, and those risks that are known are less now with the hormone therapy currently used than they were in the past. The risks can be broadly divided into relatively minor risks and psychological problems on the one hand, and remote risks of an increase of other diseases on the other hand.

Minor problems

Some women do not wish to have hormone replacement therapy on philosophical or religious grounds and regard it as 'interfering with nature'. Or they may be averse to taking regular medication. Or they may simply be glad to be rid of the problem of monthly periods. Moreover, one has to remember that many women sail through the menopause without problems and go on to a normal and long life without osteoporosis. So not all women would wish to, or would need to, take up hormone replacement treatment, even if it were freely on offer.

Other women start HRT but are bothered by the fact that they may continue to have periods and monthly breast engorgement which can be uncomfortable. The periods copy those that occurred before the menopause; if they were heavy before then they are likely to come back as heavy periods once HRT commences. Some women are worried that still having periods may mean that they are still able to have children; this is, of course, not possible as the ovaries are no longer making eggs.

Hormone replacement therapy may cause fluid retention in some women, taking the form of a temporary gain in weight and mild ankle swelling. Others develop headaches, and even vomiting. Fortunately these difficulties are not common. Although these problems sound trivial and are usually quite easily got over, they can discourage some women from continuing. The lack of an immediate benefit may mean more to them than the possibility of preventing a broken hip in 15 years' time.

More serious problems

What are the more serious risks? When hormone replacement therapy was first introduced, it was given as oestrogen alone. In the early 1970s it was found that this could cause the abnormal growth of the lining of the womb, the endometrium, and an increased risk of endometrial cancer. This is commonly called cancer of the womb. This was not as great a problem as it sounds because cancer of the womb is rare anyway. Even so, it has since been clearly shown that the addition of progestogen for at least 10 days of each monthly cycle of hormone replacement reduces, if not totally removes, the risk of this cancer. There are therefore no worries about cancer of the womb with the use of combined oestrogen-progestogen hormone replacement therapy. And if the womb has already been removed, then there is no such risk and oestrogens can safely be given without progestogen.

Another worry is whether long-term hormone replacement therapy increases the risk of breast cancer. Many millions of women have now been treated with hormone replacement therapy. At a recent meeting of the European Foundation for Osteoporosis and Bone Disease an expert panel concluded that there was no increased risk of breast cancer that should be worried about.

However, it is obviously important to be sure that there is no breast lump before starting hormone replacement therapy, either by examining the breasts or by performing a special X-ray of the breasts, known as a mammogram. Hormone replacement therapy should not be given if there has been a cancer of the breast in the past.

WHO SHOULD AND SHOULD NOT HAVE HRT?

Who should not?

The only absolute reasons for not having hormone replacement therapy are already-existing cancers of the breast or uterus. Conservative advice also suggests that hormone replacement therapy should not be given to women who have any of the factors which might stop them from using contraceptive pills; these include high blood pressure, heavy smoking, serious migraine or a history of clotting disease in the legs or elsewhere. In practice the patient and the doctor have to balance the risks of the contraceptive pill against the risks of pregnancy. In the same way for women after the menopause, you and your doctor have to balance the risks of the treatment against the risks of unprevented osteoporosis and heart attacks. These risks of treatment are not so great with hormone replacement therapy as they are with the contraceptive pill because the doses of female sex hormones used are much lower. Moreover, hormone replacement therapy – which is based on natural hormones – is given instead of, not in addition to, the natural hormones present before the menopause.

Most of the contraceptive pills contain a synthetic hormone, ethinyl oestradiol, which has a much stronger effect on the clotting process. Thrombo-embolism means blood clots forming in the veins in the legs, and in some women these blood clots get dislodged and pass to the lung, causing serious illness. A 1982 *British Medical Journal* review of all the evidence concluded that the risk of thrombo-embolism is not made greater in women after the menopause who take HRT based on natural oestrogens. Nevertheless some doctors will prefer a conservative approach unless menopausal symptoms are severe.

A subarachnoid haemorrhage is a small leak of blood around the brain. This is a very rare condition but can be fatal. Nevertheless, it is slightly more common in women taking the pill than in women not taking the pill. There is no evidence on whether it is more common in women on HRT after the menopause, but it would be unwise to treat someone with HRT who had had a subarachnoid haemorrhage in the past.

Who should have HRT?

The problem is one of deciding who is most at risk of osteoporosis. First one identifies those people for whom osteoporosis is inevitable. Then one eliminates those people for whom it is very unlikely. After that one can add up the risk factors (see page 30). A high score suggests treatment; a lower one suggests 'watch and wait – measure the density of the bones and the rate at which it is being lost.

Doctors in Denmark have evolved a fairly simple method of trying to predict who is at risk, based on a urine measurement, a blood test and an estimate of body fat from skin-fold thickness. They claim that they are about 80 per cent accurate in predicting who is a fast bone loser and who is not. Even so, a fast bone loser may be safe from developing osteoporosis if she enters maturity with good strong bones. In predicting osteoporosis the amount of bone which is present at the menopause is probably more important than the rate at which it is subsequently lost. Modern bone-density analysing machines can help but these are not yet available in all hospitals.

The decision whether or not to go on hormone replacement therapy often depends on how much a woman has read about the question, what she has heard from her friends and which symptoms of the menopause she is concerned about and wants relieved.

WHEN TO START HRT AND FOR HOW LONG?

Hormone replacement therapy will maintain bone mass if it is started within six to eight years after the menopause and it has been shown to be still effective in preventing bone loss after nine years of treatment. There are women who have been safely on hormone replacement therapy for 30 years or more and who enjoy a normal sex life in their 80s. There are others who waited for ten years after the menopause before going on hormone replacement therapy and have been shown to have some benefit as regards osteoporosis, although less than it would have been if they had started earlier. However, it is true that the longer after the menopause that hormone replacement therapy is started, the less effective it will be.

Once hormone replacement therapy is started it should be continued for at least five years, and preferably ten or more. When it is stopped the rate of loss of bone from the skeleton begins to increase but of course the loss has been permanently deferred by those five or ten years, so the skeleton will be much more likely to last for the woman's lifetime. With the average age of the menopause in British women at 52, this means that it is probably worthwhile, from the point of view of osteoporosis, starting hormone replacement therapy up to age 60 and continuing to at least age 65, and longer if well tolerated. These are conservative limits and specialist clinics are examining later starts and longer durations of treatment.

WHAT PREPARATIONS ARE AVAILABLE?

There are many chemical compounds with female sex hormone activity. It is a good rule to stick to those oestrogens which occur in nature wherever possible. Unfortunately for our convenience, the best 'natural' oestrogen, called oestradiol, if it is swallowed as a pill, is not as effective as it might be. After it is absorbed it is rapidly changed into less efficient compounds in the liver. So research has come up with derivatives of oestradiol which are more effective by mouth.

However, another answer is to give the oestradiol directly into the bloodstream through the skin, by injection, as an implanted slow-release pellet or under an adhesive patch since oestradiol can pass through normal skin.

TYPES OF HRT TREATMENT

When the womb has not been removed

Current medical opinion is that a progestogen should be given for 10 to 12 days a month, in addition to oestrogen throughout the month. This will mean a regular bleed in most women, but it will rule out any increased risk of cancer of the womb. A minor advantage is that a bleed will be completely predictable; the woman will know in advance exactly when it will take place. It will last from one to four days and will follow a fixed number of days after the date when the progestogen is stopped. In women being treated with patches or implants (see below), it is possible to control the date of the bleed. If, for example, you have a special event on the date you would normally expect a bleed and you want to be at your best, then it is possible to defer the progestogen pills so that the bleed is also deferred. However most women will be treated with one of the prepacked cyclical preparations. With Prempak and Trisequens, it is difficult to alter the date of the bleed, but it can be done with Cylcoprogynova by lengthening the seven-day gap between packs of tablets by one or two days.

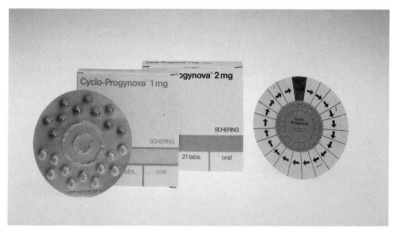

HRT pills

After a hysterectomy
For the woman who has had the womb removed, treatment is more simple. She only needs to take the oestrogen hormone, and does not need a progestogen. On theoretical grounds injections, patches or implants would be more efficient, but hundreds of thousands of women have taken oestrogens as tablets successfully.

Medicated patches
Estraderm is a medicated plaster which is changed every three to four days. It comes in three strengths, containing 25, 50 or 100 micrograms of oestradiol which is absorbed through the skin, under a waterproof adhesive plaster. For a woman who still has her uterus it is necessary to take a progestogen pill such as norethisterone acetate 1 mg for 10 to 12 days a month in addition. This is conveniently available as 'Estrapak'.

Oestradiol implants
These come in three sizes, 25, 50 or 100 mg pellets, which are slipped under the skin with a special instrument. There they slowly dissolve and may last up to a year in some women. They have to be given by a specialist clinic or by a family doctor who has had appropriate training and it is necessary to have blood tests after, say, six months to see if the pellet needs replacing.

Preparation	Type of oestrogen	Consist of	Comments
Prempak-C 28-day pack of tablets	Equine	28 maroon-coloured tablets of conjugated equine oestrogens 0.625 mg, and in addition 13 brown tablets containing progestogen (Norgestrel) 0.15 mg taken from day 17 to day 28.	Continuous oestrogen. Intermittent progestogen. Equine oestrogens have a longer effect and withstand digestion better than oestradiol.
Cycloprogynova 21-day pack of tablets	Human	11 beige-coloured tablets of oestradiol valerate 1.0 mg followed by 10 brown mixed tablets of oestradiol valerate 1.0 mg plus a progestogen (Levonorgestrol) 0.25 mg	Discontinuous oestrogen. Intermittent progestogen. No tablet is taken from day 22 to day 28, after which the next pack is started.
Trisequens 28-day pack of tablets	Human	12 blue mixed tablets of oestradiol 2 mg plus oestriol 1 mg, followed by 10 white mixed tablets of oestradiol 2 mg plus oestriol 1 mg plus norethisterone acetate 1 mg, followed by 6 red mixed tablets containing oestradiol 1.0 mg plus oestriol 0.5 mg.	Continuous oestrogen. Intermittent progestogen. Convenient dispenser makes it difficult to make mistakes.

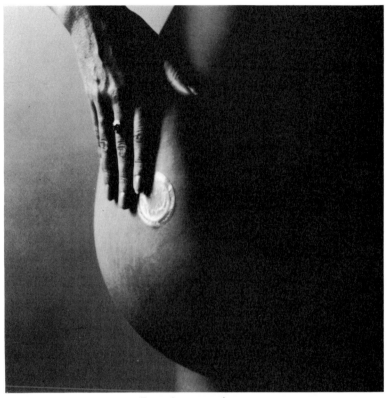

Estraderm patch

As with the patches, the advantage of a one-shot treatment is reduced by the need to take a progestogen pill for 10 to 12 days a month if you have not had a hysterectomy.

Other methods
Oestrogens can be absorbed from ointments, gels, or vaginal pessaries but it is more difficult to control the dose

HRT and calcium
Calcium supplements on their own cannot substitute for lack of oestrogen; without oestrogen the bones cannot take up calcium as they should, but with oestrogen the calcium can go into the bones. So calcium treatment can supplement oestrogen treatment but not substitute for it. However it has been found that, by giving calcium with oestrogen, only half the dose of oestrogen is needed.

BEFORE STARTING HRT

It is good practice for the doctor to give you a thorough check-up first, including a pelvic examination to exclude any problem such as fibroids in the womb which might be made to grow if HRT is given. It should also include a breast examination or possibly a mammogram, and the blood pressure should be checked. The doctor may also ask you about things which in his or her opinion may make HRT inadvisable.

For you it is necessary to plan to take HRT for many years, and not give up because you 'can't be bothered' or because it seems inconvenient. HRT costs money and, by a quirk of the National Health Service, the combined packs of tablets are charged as two prescriptions, despite the fact that avoiding costly hip fractures in later life will save the NHS much more than the cost of drugs. Implants certainly, and patches preferably, need to be monitored by blood tests to see if the dose is enough.

Remember, also, that HRT is not a magic drug for rejuvenation; you will still get older year by year. What it will do is put off those changes caused by hormone lack after the menopause, changes which are not a necessary and inevitable part of the ageing process.

HOW SHOULD HRT BE SUPERVISED?

It is very important that hormone replacement therapy should not be given unless the patient has had time to have full medical counselling so that she understands the problems and the necessary precautions. She must realise that to prevent osteoporosis, long-term treatment is necessary – we really ought to talk about supervised hormone replacement therapy, SHRT, rather than just HRT.

A woman should also have a full examination, including pelvic, breast and blood pressure examination, every year preferably, or at least every second year whilst on treatment. Certain centres have bone-density machines which can tell how the treatment is working and whether it needs to be adjusted. Any bleeding other than the monthly period should be notified to the doctor supervising treatment and it may then be necessary to take a sample of the lining of the womb. Nowadays this does not always mean a general anaesthetic.

8

PREVENTION IN THE ELDERLY

We all lose bone as we age, so inevitably there will be some degree of osteoporosis in the elderly. Most of this could have been prevented by hormone replacement therapy (see previous chapter), but once it has taken place it can only be reversed to a very limited extent, and only in some people. One is therefore restricted to trying to prevent any further loss and, most importantly, to prevent the consequence of osteoporosis – a fracture. Such fractures are usually related to falls and it is important to understand why the elderly fall, and how falls and other untoward events which are likely to lead to fractures, can be prevented, thus avoiding the consequences of osteoporosis in this age group.

PREVENTING FURTHER BONE LOSS

In the elderly (usually taken as men and women over 70) the main lines of prevention of osteoporosis are just as important as in younger groups:

- Diet – including sufficient calcium and a trace of flouride.
- Exercise.
- A continuation of hormone replacement therapy for some women.

Diet

Calcium and Vitamin D An elderly intestine is less efficient than a young one in absorbing calcium from the diet. So an

71

elderly person should be taking in more calcium in the diet to compensate for this. The British Recommended Daily Allowance (RDA) of calcium of 500 mg a day is too low for elderly people; 1500 mg a day is nearer the mark. Irrespective of this, vitamin D is needed for absorption of calcium into the body. Most of our vitamin D comes from exposure of the skin to the sun's ultraviolet rays, and many elderly people do not go out in the sun, especially in winter. They may live indoors behind glass, travel in cars behind glass, and glass does not let ultraviolet light through. Experiments with young submariners have shown that, on a normal diet, it only takes three months of being shut away from the sun to bring about a drastic reduction in the rate of absorption of calcium.

There are various solutions to this problem, the easiest being, of course, to take more vitamin D in the diet – not much is needed, only 400 international units a day. Much more than this may even make osteoporosis worse. Another solution is to fit windows or conservatories with plastic transparent glazing which allows ultraviolet light to pass through. Strip lights which have a 'full daylight spectrum' can also be fitted. These emit ultraviolet light just as the sun does.

Much of this has been known for a long time. Nevertheless a recent Medical Research Council Survey of a Harrow hospital disclosed that many patients admitted had been living on a deficient diet. However, it was those who never got out in the sun who developed weak bones.

Exercise

Older people need to keep mobile. Just as in younger people, exercise is needed to keep bones strong when you get older. Research has shown that you only have to walk a few miles a week to reduce the loss of bone from the skeleton. Swimming is good at maintaining mobility and muscle but is not as good for the skeleton; weight-bearing exercise such as walking is best.

A simple exercise programme for the mobile elderly is shown on pages 103–13.

There are obvious difficulties with this for some who have already lost mobility. If frail elderly people are encouraged to do such exercises they are, of course, more in danger of falling and great care must be taken. Nevertheless, the picture now is of too many elderly people who have lost their mobility spending nearly all the evening of their lives in a bed or chair when, with a little encouragement and help, either by provision of walking aids, by adaptation of their homes, or by help from the caring professions and relatives, they could be kept mobile and their bones kept stronger. Often it is loss of confidence rather than loss of ability that stops them walking. In particular they lose their confidence in going down stairs even though they are usually still capable of doing so. The provision of an extra handrail may restore that confidence. Similarly, many elderly people rely on well-known furniture to support them as they move about the house. If someone 'tidies up' and moves the furniture they may fall. The provision of handrails – in passageways, in toilets and bathrooms and on doors – so that there is something that is easy to hold on to helps improve mobility. The various walking aids, from a stick to a frame, can also provide vital support to prevent falling. A little imagination will often suggest other ways in which mobility can be helped for those who are insecure and unsure of their footing.

A home visit from an occupational therapist may be needed – they are trained to spot practical home adaptations which would be helpful and to advise on how these can be done. They or a physiotherapist can decide if the elderly person would be helped by some walking aid and arrange for this to be supplied.

Hormone replacement therapy
Hormone replacement therapy will almost certainly prevent further loss of bone from the skeleton in women, at whatever age it is started, and it is recommended by some doctors. The longer after menopause, however, the less acceptable is the likely return of periods and other symptoms occasionally associated with this treatment, as outlined in the previous chapter. If one has had an hysterectomy then this form of treatment might be reasonable to consider.

FALLS

More than one in three elderly people will have a minor fall each year. Such falls lead to broken bones more frequently than in the young, and the frequency rises very steeply in the very old. The frequency of fractures is further increased in winter because of wet or icy pavements. The elderly are admitted to hospital more often than are younger people following a fall; when people over 60 attend hospital as a result of a fall, 60 per cent of them are found to have a fracture, many of these in the hip.

The risk of death from such a fall is quite significant. In 1982 in the United States, 11,600 deaths followed falls, 70 per cent of which occurred in the elderly. The rate rose rapidly over the age of 65; a quarter of people over 90 who had fallen and attended hospital died, while over half of those who had a hip fracture over the age of 90 died. One study found that the inability to walk out of doors unaided was the best predictor of the risk of falling.

Many of these falls can be prevented by proper attention to the factors which cause them – the provision of adequate grab rails, walking aids, lighting and the avoidance of over-medication which might cause confusion or drops in blood pressure.

There are numerous causes of falls in the elderly. These can be broadly divided into those due to the elderly person themselves (internal causes) and those causes due to their environment (external causes) although quite often both kinds of risk are present.

Internal causes

As one gets older there is a general deterioration of many functions; for example, balance, muscular strength and eyesight are all poorer. If the elderly do fall, they are less able to break the impact of the fall because they are weaker, they react more slowly and they have less protective muscle and fat. Some illnesses affect mobility and stability, for example arthritis and Parkinson's disease. Confinement to bed for a few days with any illness such as flu or pneumonia is often followed by some loss of balance and co-ordination, so that when the elderly person gets up and about again, he or she is more tottery and more liable to fall.

Blackouts account for about one-quarter of all falls in the elderly and may occur for several reasons. Most commonly they are the result of changes in blood pressure or heart rate. In elderly people the pulse rate is sometimes not stable – the heart may beat irregularly once or twice, or 'miss a beat' for a

Causes of falls in the over 70's

General problems
    Poor balance
    Poor gait
    Weakness
    Poor vision
    Slow reflexes

Specific problems
    Arthritis
    Strokes (cerebrovascular disease)
    Parkinson's disease
    Ménière's disease
    Cataracts and retinal degeneration
    Blackouts
        low blood pressure
        irregular heart beat (arrhythmias)
        temporary lack of blood to the brain
          (transient ischaemic attacks)
        epileptic fits
        low blood sugar
    Drugs
        sleeping pills
        blood pressure pills
        diabetic pills
    Alcohol

In the home
    Slippery surfaces
    Uneven pavements
    Loose rugs
    Bad weather
    Tripping over pets, children's toys, etc.

few seconds – and during that time not enough blood will be going to the brain. This causes sudden dizziness or loss of consciousness, followed by a fall. Sometimes the main arteries carrying blood to the brain are partly blocked and if the blood pressure drops a little there is the same result – not enough oxygen gets to the brain, dizziness or unconsciousness follow and the person falls. In other elderly people the regulation of the blood pressure is at fault, so standing up suddenly – getting out of bed, standing up after a meal, getting up suddenly out of a hot bath – may be followed by a drop in blood pressure and a fall. This can also happen in the night when getting up to go to the toilet.

In diabetics, a low blood sugar can cause loss of consciousness, while in others unconsciousness follows a cough. And there are many other less common causes.

Some of these drop attacks can be indirectly the result of treatment that is being taken for other problems. For example, treatment for high blood pressure, if overdone, will be followed by too low a blood pressure and this may lead to a drop attack. The use of diuretics ('water pills') may have the same effect. Alcohol may be more intoxicating in the elderly than in the young, and sometimes old people are taking large amounts of alcohol, unbeknown to others.

Perhaps the greatest hazard is from drugs given for depression, anxiety or sleeplessness. These can lead to drowsiness, confusion, disorientation and poor balance, especially if there are other drugs given at the same time. With many of the treatments, this is a particular problem during the night and first thing in the morning.

External causes
External factors contribute to about one-third of all falls, although they are commonly combined with internal factors; for example, poor lighting and a loose rug may be combined with poor eyesight. Common external causes of fractures are steep stairs, slippery surfaces such as wet floors and icy pavements, loose rugs, uneven paving stones, poor footwear, worn footrubbers on sticks or crutches, and inadequate lighting.

Unfamiliar surroundings frequently lead to elderly people falling. When grandma goes to visit her grandchildren, what should be a joyful family reunion may turn into a tragedy when, groping her way to the unfamiliar lavatory at night, she falls over some discarded toy; or in the daytime she gets up from a chair and trips over a pet dog. Three-quarters of all falls occur indoors in the bedroom or living room, often merely on getting out of bed or out of a chair.

9

HOW EFFECTIVE
ARE TREATMENTS FOR
OSTEOPOROSIS?

This is really only a small part of the question 'How does one measure the effectiveness of any treatment in medicine?'

For some conditions it is easy to show the benefit of a treatment. Take, for example, the condition tuberculous meningitis (inflammation of the coverings of the brain caused by the tuberculosis bacteria). It used to be a killer; no one with it recovered. Today it can be treated with antibiotics. For such a condition, the survivors demonstrate how effective treatment is.

At the other end of the scale, there are illnesses that will get better whatever we do. In these, any treatment which is tried appears to be followed by a cure. Consider the common cold. Take no treatment and it can take up to a fortnight to get better. Take large doses of vitamin C pills and you will be better in two weeks. If you have a lot of faith in vitamin C, it will probably be hard to convince you that the treatment had nothing to do with the cure.

In the middle are those conditions, like osteoporosis and arthritis, which over the years are slowly progressive but which, from one month to another may show surprising ups and downs – at some times these may be more painful than at others. You usually seek help when you are in a 'down', and the chances are that before long you will be in an 'up'; the result is therefore that whatever treatment you get given, unless it is positively harmful, will appear to have helped you. If the treatment given was 'non-scientific' the healer will feel he has gone a good job and earned his fee, and you will no doubt give him the credit and be grateful.

The 'scientific' doctor, however, has to do more than that. He has to show that if the treatment was repeated in large groups of osteoporosis sufferers, more of them would improve than would have been expected to from chance alone. Moreover he would have to show that any seeming side effects were also more than would be expected by chance or coincidence.

TESTING A TREATMENT

To test a treatment for osteoporosis (or for any complaint, for that matter) we have to take a sufficiently large group of sufferers and divide them into two groups by a method, such as tossing a coin, which makes it a matter of chance into which of the two groups any one individual is placed. Nowadays it is not done by tossing coins – a computer will do the job of random allocation – but the principle is the same. Then one group of patients is given the new treatment and the other group is either given a 'placebo' (a dummy tablet that looks like the active treatment but in fact has no drug in it) or is given the previously best available treatment, again preferably dressed up to be undistinguishable from the test drug. Someone not directly concerned with the tests keeps the code which says which osteoporosis sufferer is on which treatment. So the patient does not know which treatment he or she is having and, in an ideal test, the doctor or whoever is assessing the new drug does not know either. (If anything goes amiss for a patient the code can of course be broken, the doctor can find out what treatment is being used in that particular case, and the patient can then be withdrawn from the trial if necessary.)

The designer of this sort of trial is known as a medical statistician. Apart from organising true randomisation of sufferers to one treatment or another, his other problems include deciding with the doctor in charge how long a trial should go on and what are the best things to measure, so as to decide whether the treatment is working.

From the point of view of the osteoporosis sufferer, the most important measure is the amount of pain relief. But, although it sounds hard hearted, from the point of view of the medical scientist pain is not a good measure. Pain is extraordinarily variable and so are the ways people react to it. Think for example, of a headache. Most people get a headache from time to time. Such headaches are not serious, soon recover, and are more of a nuisance than a disaster. But think how a headache is often described – not just a headache, but a 'splitting headache' or a 'dreadful headache' or 'it's killing me'. The words people use do not match up to the severity of the pain.

What we are driving at here is that doctors, in their role as medical scientists, try to measure what are known as 'objective changes'.

Large-scale trials

With some treatments, such as different types of HRT, the advantages of one drug over another may be small. Even so they may be worthwhile. But if the advantage is small, it may take very large groups of patients to show it. To get over this a European Foundation for Research into Osteoporosis and Bone Disease has been set up so that medical researchers can pool their knowledge and resources.

How long should a clinical trial last?

This depends on the rate at which improvement is expected to occur, and has usually been found out beforehand on one or two patients. Oestrogens produce a measurable change in bone density fairly quickly, so a clinical trial of a new form of oestrogen might take six months. But calcium treatment, for example in the osteoporosis which occurs as a complication of corticosteroid treatment, works very slowly, and several years may be needed to produce a really convincing result.

The testing of treatments in osteoporosis is thus a very slow process. Changes in bone take a long time to occur and the best machines cannot show the effects in less than 6 to 12 months. Many of the treatments only have a slow and slight effect so that measurements must be made over a few years, especially if you want to see whether fractures are prevented. To try and get a quicker answer as to whether a treatment might work and that it is worth investing in the necessary long-term studies, you can measure the levels in the blood and urine of the breakdown products of some bone tissues. If bone is being protected, these breakdown products are reduced.

And this is not the end of the story. Some treatments 'work' at first, but the body then gets used to them and the effect wears off, even if treatment is continued.

OUTCOME MEASURE IN OSTEOPOROSIS

It would be very nice if one could use bone strength as a measure of osteoporosis. In a testing laboratory, the strength of any material can easily be measured by placing a rod made from the material across two supports, then applying increasing weights to the middle until it bends or breaks. Fortunately or unfortunately, there is no way of doing this in the living subject. The nearest we can get to it is to measure bone density, and assume that a bone which has the greatest density has the greatest strength. This is broadly true but there are exceptions. For example in the condition known as 'marble-bone disease', bones are exceedingly dense on X-ray but they are also exceptionally brittle. The same is true if large amounts of fluoride are taken – more than are used in the treatment of osteoporosis; the bones become denser but they also fracture more easily.

Fracture rate

In fact the only true way of estimating bone strength in life is by the fracture rate. One has to take very large groups of osteoporosis sufferers and follow them for a number of years, recording how many fractures occur in each group. If one group of patients is being treated with, say, calcium, and a second group with calcium and oestrogen, and the first group gets twice as many fractures as the second group, then it is reasonable to suppose that the combination of calcium and oestrogen is the better treatment. Just how reasonable this conclusion is can also be put into numbers by the medical statistician. He can say whether or not a difference between the two groups is likely to have arisen purely by chance; if the difference is unlikely to have arisen by chance, he will call it a statistically significant difference.

Using the fracture rate as an outcome measure, it has been shown that women who take a large amount of calcium in their food throughout life get fewer hip fractures than women who take only a little calcium. It has also been used to show that women who do not have a normal trace of fluoride in their water supply have an increased risk of hip fractures, and, more recently, that women who are taking HRT can reduce their risk of hip fractures by as much as two-thirds.

X-rays

X-rays are not much good at measuring bone density, as a third of the density is lost before it shows on the X-ray. But X-rays do show bone structure, and if you have osteoporosis then the bones in the palm of the hand, the metacarpals (and the corresponding bones in the feet), show structural changes. These are all tubular bones, and the hard outer part of the bone, the cortex, gets thinner in osteoporosis, and the inner empty space gets wider. Doctors can measure these changes accurately, and by dividing the width of the cortex by the width of the whole bone can come up with a number which is a measurement of osteoporosis. This method has been used extensively as it is inexpensive and simple to do.

Another change that can be seen on X-rays concerns the trabecular (spongy) bone in the hip. In a normal bone this shows up strongly but it becomes less and less clear with osteoporosis. A series of standard patterns has been adopted, and the appearance of the sufferer's bone is matched up with these. This is called the Singh index, after the person who first devised it. It has been used in large studies of elderly women brought to hospital after a fall. Those women who had fractured a hip had a lower Singh index, i.e. worse osteoporosis, than similar women X-rayed after a fall who were found not to have fractured a hip.

Measuring spinal osteoporosis

Testing treatments for spinal osteoporosis is not so easy. Fractures may be painless and go unnoticed. To see the effect of any treatment, before-and-after X-rays will be needed. The number of crushed vertebrae can then be counted, their loss of height measured or their change in shape scored.

Alternatively, body height can be measured to see if the treatment stops a spinal osteoporosis sufferer from shrinking. Again, though, there are some difficulties as the osteoporotic spine does not shrink at a steady rate but does so slowly at first, then relatively rapidly. And shrinkage does not go on indefinitely; there is a limit beyond which, however severe, an osteoporotic spine cannot shrink further.

When patients with osteoporotic spines come to a clinic for bone diseases, their height will usually be measured. But some will come early, when the shrinkage has just started, and others will come late, when it is unlikely that they will shrink any more. Consequently any treatment given to the last group would appear to be successful if it was measured by how well it stopped the 'shrinking'. The method can be used, but it again means that large groups of patients have to be compared.

Measuring bone density

There are now machines that will measure bone density, the amount of calcium in a certain volume of bone, although at present few hospitals in Great Britain have these machines. They can measure bone density in the forearm (single photon absorptiometers) or in the hip and spine (dual photon absorptiometers and computerised tomography). These machines work by measuring the amount of nuclear or X-ray energy that the bone prevents from passing through itself.

HOW DOES THIS AFFECT THE OSTEOPOROSIS SUFFERER?

At present there is no perfect treatment for established osteoporosis. So the hunt is on for something better. This may be something quite new, or it may be a combination of existing treatments. Because of this, many specialist centres for bone diseases undertake clinical trials, and you may be asked to take part in one.

If this occurs, you should expect a full explanation of what is happening and what the doctors are trying to find out. Accept the invitation if you can; not only is this the only way to discover better treatments, but you will also probably become one of the best-looked after patients in the hospital. As well as being measured to test the benefit of the treatment, you will also be carefully observed and asked to report any possible side effects of treatment. At the end of the clinical trial you should expect to be told what drug it was you helped test, what the results were and if these were beneficial, and whether the drug has been or will be released for general use.

10

TREATMENTS FOR OSTEOPOROSIS

Once the hard mineral is lost from bones, there is very little that can be done to put it back. That is why the emphasis in this book has been on prevention. We hope that it will not be always so – intense medical research is going on today to uncover the secrets of living bone, and it is certain that a way of restoring lost mineral and strength to osteoporotic bones will be found eventually.

For those people whose osteoporosis has been discovered by chance before a fracture has occurred and for those people who have already had an osteoporotic fracture of a limb bone which has now healed, treatment consists of preventing things from getting worse and avoiding the risks which may lead to falls and accidents. For those people who have the mainly spinal form of osteoporosis, treatment is also a question of adapting to the altered body shape and posture and treating the complications these may produce in the chest and abdomen.

Treatments to prevent worsening of the osteoporosis will have no immediate benefits; for example, they will not immediately relieve pain – something else will be needed for that. The purpose of these treatments is to prevent further fractures over the remaining years.

TREATMENTS TO PREVENT OSTEOPOROSIS

Calcium

The calcium-containing crystals of bone mineral in normal bones are packed along the fibres of collagen, but the brittle bones of osteoporosis have not only too little calcium in them, they have also too little collagen. It is collagen which forms the framework or 'scaffolding' of bone. This means that until new scaffolding can be made, there is not enough room for new bone mineral to be laid down. It all takes time.

Because of this, once osteoporosis is established there is no immediately obvious effect of calcium treatment on the bones or on their liability to fracture. This has even led some scientists to suggest that calcium has nothing to do with osteoporosis – forgetting all the evidence that lack of calcium in the past has been a major contributing cause of osteoporosis and the evidence that people who live in places where their diet contains plenty of calcium get fewer fractures than similar people who live in places where the diet is low in calcium.

Following on from the careful studies of a group of doctors in Omaha, USA, it is now known that, to protect themselves against osteoporosis, women should be regularly taking about 1 g (1,000 mg) of calcium daily before the menopause and 1.5 g (1,500 mg) after the menopause. First one has to make a rough guess as to how much calcium is already in the diet. This is easy (see page 49) – it often depends on whether the person concerned takes milk regularly. If so she will be getting about 700 mg of calcium a day in each pint. However, most people these days make a pint of milk last two days and on average, from all food sources, surveys show that women generally get only between 400 and 700 mg of calcium per day. This means giving a calcium supplement of 500 mg before the menopause and about 1,000 mg after it.

Many calcium supplements are available under the National Health Service, and many others can be bought in chemists and healthfood shops. However, you should ensure that they do contain a useful amount of calcium. Remember that after the menopause a daily total of about 1.5 g calcium should be taken in the diet and by the use of these supplements if necessary.

Should we buy calcium tablets with added vitamin D? The answer is generally no. For uncomplicated osteoporosis vitamin D is not helpful; it merely puts up the expense. Getting outside in daylight for a few hours a day, and eating some fish will provide plenty of this vitamin.

It is true that not all calcium preparations are absorbed equally from the gut but the differences are small and do not matter. On general principles it is probably better to take as

Calcium Supplements Prescribable under the NHS

Proprietory name	Generic name	Tablet size (mg)	Calcium content per tablet (mg)	No. of tablets to provide approximately		Comment
				600 mg calcium	1,100 mg calcium	
Ossopan 800	Hydroxyapatite compound	830	178	4	6	Bone mineral from young beef bones. Also available as powder
Sandocal	Calcium lactate gluconate	3,080	400	1½	3	Dissolves in water. Also contains sodium and potassium
Titralac	Calcium carbonate	420	105	6	11	May also be bought without prescription
Calcichew	Calcium carbonate	1,200	500	1	2	

Doctors are permitted to prescribe calcium gluconate BP and calcium lactate BP tablets but these contain too little calcium to be practical.

much as possible of the calcium required in the diet. Milk is the most important source. For people who want to slim, skimmed milks are available, as well as fortified skimmed milks which contain extra calcium. Since the war the consumption of milk per person has declined from 4½ to 2½ pints a week in Britain, mainly because of worries about too much milk fat causing obesity or heart disease. This may well have something to do with the increase in the frequency of osteoporosis over the same period.

Fluoride

People who live in districts where the water contains an excess of fluoride (5 parts per million or more) get dense bone and stiffened spines. People who live in districts where the water supply is deficient in fluoride (½ part per million or less) get weak bones and poor teeth. Giving fluoride alone to people who already have osteoporosis makes their bones denser but not necessarily stronger, unless plenty of calcium is also given.

The usual dose of fluoride is 40 mg per day given in two doses and taken with food. The preparation is sodium fluoride and it comes in 20 mg film-coated tablets or in 10 and 20 mg capsules. It can only be prescribed by a doctor in these doses. However, there are 1 mg size tablets which can be obtained over the counter and which are ostensibly available for giving to children in low fluoride districts in order to help protect their teeth, but they will also help protect the children in those districts from osteoporosis in later life.

The small doses of fluoride used for prevention are generally very well tolerated and produce no side effects. The higher doses used for treatment of established osteoporosis, in the range of 40 mg per day or more, can upset some people, though. The indigestion and digestive problems caused by taking fluoride are usually temporary and get better, despite continuing with the treatment. However, some people also get rheumatic symptoms; their limbs become painful and stiff and their joints may even swell occasionally. This usually means that the treatment is not going to be tolerated, even if persisted with. These effects are more common with the higher doses. Some doctors and specialist centres give doses of 80 mg or more per day, based on theoretical grounds. However, it is probably better to use lower doses and wait a bit longer for the benefits.

Vitamin D

Vitamin D is essential for life and particularly essential for the formation of good bones and the efficient absorption of calcium from the gut into the bloodstream. However, up to 90 per cent of vitamin D is made by the body in the skin, so adding vitamin D to the diet (which usually contains some anyway) is seldom necessary. Vitamin D, made by the action of ultraviolet light on substances in the skin, has a safety feature; if you already have enough, your skin stops making any more. But vitamin D that you swallow ready-made has no such safety feature, so if you take more than you need you store some of it in your liver. This helps you get over the days in winter when not much ultraviolet light from the sun is available. Once the store is full, however, and you still go on swallowing vitamin D, you actually risk making osteoporosis worse.

Vitamin D deficiency still does occur in some women who for ethnic or cultural reasons, cover up their skin with black clothing, and who fail to expose any of their skin to whatever sunlight is available. This is particularly true if they spend most of their time indoors or in cars, behind glass. Elderly persons who are confined to their houses because of arthritis or some other infirmity and who never get out in the sun are also at risk of vitamin D deficiency. Vitamin D deficiency can be prevented by taking 10 micrograms (400 units) of calciferol daily. There is no danger of overdosage with this. However, larger doses of vitamin D can be harmful and should only be taken under medical supervision for special reasons. Doctors usually prescribe one tablet of 'calcium with vitamin D'. The amount of calcium in this is very little but the amount of vitamin D is enough. Alternatively, multivitamin tablets are available which give a supplement of several sorts of vitamins and minerals, and one a day of these provides enough vitamin D.

There are several kinds of vitamin D with different chemical names, and vitamin D is also sold as cod liver oil or as halibut liver oil capsules. They are all activated in the liver and kidneys into the final essential form. So if you are buying vitamin D preparations do it on the number of international units they contain, not the weight in milligrams or micrograms.

Calcitonin

Calcitonin is a hormone made by the thyroid gland, the job of which is to suppress the action of osteoclasts – the cells which remove bone prior to the action of osteoblasts, the cells which build bone (see page 8). In some kinds of osteoporosis, where the osteoclasts are over-active, calcitonin treatment stops bone loss and may even cause bone gain. This gain has not yet been shown to last for more than 18 months and overall the results of giving calcitonin are not as as yet very impressive, but more research is being done.

There are disadvantages to calcitonin. It is very expensive and it must be given by injection at least three times a week. However, newer cheaper ways to make it have been developed, and it may soon be available as a nasal spray which would make taking it much easier. Some patients are sensitive to it, giving them problems with nausea and occasionally vomiting. At present it is mainly given in specialist centres as part of studies of treatments for osteoporosis.

Anabolic steroids

These are the steroids which are derived from male sex hormones and which athletes use (illegally) in order to build up their muscles and their muscle strength. They can also build up bone strength. The common preparations given are stanozolol, usually given as 2 mg three times a week by mouth for three in every four weeks together with 1 g of calcium daily. An alternative is injections of another anabolic steroid dissolved in oil, called nandralone decanoate, which is given at three-weekly intervals, 25 mg at a time, usually for a limited number of weeks.

While undoubtedly effective, particularly over the course of one to two years, the results of stanozolol usually wear off in time. The treatment is somewhat expensive and the side effects may include masculinisation, with growth of moustache hair. However, anabolic steroids may be particularly useful in helping recovery from osteoporosis-related fractures.

Parathyroid hormone

This is not now used for osteoporosis, but may be helpful in certain combinations with other drugs as a way to wake up the bone cells so that they can be stimulated to make more bone.

Bisphosphonates (or diphosphonates)

These are drugs developed from the water-softening agents added to washing-machine powders. They act on bone mineral crystals in two ways: they can stop small crystals from forming; and they can protect larger crystals from being dissolved. Which action occurs most depends on the chemical composition of the bisphosphonate and on the dose. There are now a number of careful studies showing that, at least in the short term, they can protect bones against loss of density, but they have not yet been shown to reduce the risk of fracture.

Other drugs

So much effort is now being put into discovering new drugs for osteoporosis that by the time this book is published the above list will probably be incomplete.

Drug companies which undertake research have millions of drugs whose names and properties are stored in their computers. When looking for an osteoporosis drug they will select out of these millions some that have known actions on calcium, or on some process known to be related to bone formation. These are called candidate drugs. The next step is to check that they are not toxic, and then to test them in experimental osteoporosis. Birds which lay eggs (and lose calcium in the eggshells) get osteoporosis if they do not get enough calcium in their feed. Hen turkeys are usually chosen, as they are large birds which can more easily be studied by X-ray or bone-density measurements. Out of the many candidate drugs, one or two may show some promise for human use. After more elaborate safety and toxicity tests, these may be tested in normal human volunteers and only after that in osteoporosis sufferers.

PAIN RELIEF

In its early stages osteoporosis is completely painless, and in the form which mainly affects the limbs it remains painless until a fracture occurs. That of course can be very painful. Strong pain-relieving drugs such as morphine may be needed, because even with the best of intentions, and the best designed ambulances, getting a patient to a hospital jogs the fracture and causes severe pain. Some doctors who have learnt the necessary skills inject a local anaesthetic into the fracture line.

This produces rapid, although short-lived, relief of pain, and may make all the difference between a comfortable and an excruciatingly painful transfer to hospital, especially for those with hip fractures.

For the spinal form of osteoporosis the acute vertebral collapse fracture can also be extremely painful and may require very strong painkillers, although the pain usually settles after a few weeks. In some people spinal osteoporosis produces chronic back pain, due to the stooped posture causing muscle spasm and putting an increased stress on other parts of the spine, particularly the neck. Pain relief is then needed. Paracetamol is an extremely safe pain-relieving drug providing not more than eight tablets (4 g in total) are taken in a day. You do not 'get used to it' and it is not addictive. If you are in pain, there is no benefit in rationing yourself in these tablets. Paracetamol is found in several painkiller tablets in combination with other drugs, such as in co-proxamol and co-codamol. Codeine-containing painkiller tablets for pain may constipate.

Another group of painkiller tablets are called non-steroidal anti-inflammatory drugs (NSAIDs). These work in a way similar to aspirin and are effective in relieving pain. They occasionally irritate the stomach, causing indigestion and rarely an ulcer. They should be avoided if you already have these stomach problems.

There are non-drug ways of relieving back pain. We do not recommend manipulation of the spine – it will already be fragile and commonsense would say avoid forceful movements. Acupuncture or an electrical device, TENS, which works in a similar way, are sometimes effective at relieving chronic pain. Corsets of the kind that are often used for ordinary back pain are not to be recommended in osteoporosis; it is usually the upper spine that is affected and if you splint this with a corset, then breathing is restricted, and if the low back is supported, then the stomach is compressed causing discomfort and the inability to eat a full meal.

TREATMENT OF ACUTE SPINAL
CRUSH-FRACTURE SYNDROME

In brief this consists of putting the sufferer on bed rest or rest in a chair for as brief a period as is tolerated, and giving pain-relieving drugs which may include strong painkillers derived from morphine until the severe pain settles. It includes in some instances giving anabolic steroids to speed up the fracture-healing process and it includes advice not to use spinal supports or braces unless life is absolutely intolerable without them.

Most spinal crush fractures get much less painful within about three weeks, enabling the patient to get around again, perhaps a little shorter in height, but nevertheless not immobilised in bed.

EXERCISE

Lack of mobility causes loss of bone and leads to osteoporosis. Plenty of physical activity whilst the skeleton is developing results in denser stronger bones. Exercise after middle age, after the menopause, reduces the loss of bone that you would expect from the skeleton. This only needs to be a small amount, such as walking for three hours a week – you do not have to take up jogging.

It is important to do exercises that do not increase your risk of falling. Swimming is good at maintaining your muscle and general fitness, but is not so good for the skeleton. The best exercises for the bones are those that put the weight of the body on the skeleton. Walking is the simplest and best exercise.

SURGERY

The chief contribution of surgery is in the setting of fractures of the limb bones and in replacement of the joint (arthroplasty) for fractures of the hip. Although thinned, osteoporotic bones heal normally. It is sometimes helpful to remove the lower ribs in patients with spinal osteoporosis where the height has decreased so much that the ribs are pressing painfully on the pelvis. Usually only one side needs this treatment.

Some patients with very severe spinal osteoporosis find that their heads come right down forward on their chests and may get set in this position. At some stage in the future it may be possible to alter the angle of the neck so that it is possible to see forwards but this is as yet experimental surgery; only to be tried in very serious problems where life is otherwise intolerable.

DRUGS WHICH INTERFERE WITH OSTEOPOROSIS TREATMENT

Corticosteroids

These are the worst offenders. Not only do they cause osteoporosis, but they also reduce the effectiveness of treatments for osteoporosis. It may not be possible to come off them, but every effort should be made to ensure that you are taking as little as necessary for as short a time as possible. You should not alter the dose without your doctor's knowledge and agreement as this can upset the illness for which you are taking them.

Sometimes reducing the dose is better achieved by putting small doses directly into painful joints in arthritis, or by using a corticosteroid inhaler in asthma, or a prednisolone enema in colitis.

Fluoride and calcium together

Taking fluoride and calcium at the same time reduces their effectiveness because insoluble compounds are formed. They should be spaced, say by taking the calcium at breakfast and the fluoride with midday and evening meals.

Taking too much salt

We normally only need about 2 g of salt (sodium chloride) a day. The more you take, the more comes out in the urine. Unfortunately it tends to draw out calcium with it. Salt cheeses, salt meats like ham, tinned meats and packet soups are the worst offenders. The effect is not very important, and we do not suggest you 'black' these good foods and avoid them altogether – just keep the amounts you eat down.

It is a good idea to stick to unprocessed food, avoiding adding salt to cooking recipes and avoid sprinkling salt on your meals.

Things which make for acid urine

If you eat only vegetables you will have an alkaline urine. If you eat only meat and fish, your urine will be acid. This is because the latter foods contain sulphur and phosphorus, two substances which are essential to our body cells but which in excess are turned into acids which, when they come out in the urine, draw calcium with them. It is thought that this may be one of the reasons why vegetarians get less osteoporosis than meat-eaters. Again we do not suggest that you cut out all fish and meat, but it would be worthwhile having, say, one or two meat-free days a week.

Some bottled cola drinks contain phosphoric acid to give them a sharp taste. This also makes the urine acid.

Aluminium-hydroxide-based antacids

If you are an indigestion sufferer, you may need to take antacids. Many of these are based on aluminium hydroxide, which neutralises stomach acids. Unfortunately they bind to phosphorus, and the phosphorus has to come from the calcium phosphate in the bones, taking out the calcium with it. If you do need an antacid, switch to one that contains calcium carbonate.

'Water pills' (diuretics)

These are used to encourage the kidneys to make more urine, and are useful to relieve fluid retention and congestion in heart disease, liver disease or kidney disease. They also are used to reduce blood pressure. However, they do cause the kidney to excrete more calcium. The effect is not great, and can be overcome by taking an extra calcium pill.

If you are one of those people who get fluid retention and ankle swelling with hormone replacement therapy, you may need a diuretic temporarily to get over this. Do not stop taking a diuretic which you have been prescribed without seeing your doctor. You are unlikely to have been given them without a good and serious reason.

TREATMENT FOR ASSOCIATED MEDICAL PROBLEMS

In spinal osteoporosis there is a tendency to develop other medical problems.

Shortness of breath

This may develop because there is less room in the chest after the spine shrinks. It can be helped to some extent by physiotherapy directed at breathing exercises.

Indigestion and regurgitation

Because there is less room in the abdomen there is sometimes the problem of regurgitation of acid stomach contents into the gullet, giving pain. Sometimes all or part of the stomach moves upwards (hiatus hernia).

Antacids (indigestion mixtures) that contain alginates can be very helpful here. Avoid stooping forwards, for example in gardening or when leaning over a wash basin or fire grate after a meal; stooping increases the tendency for the stomach and its contents to be pushed back up into the chest. Sleep with the head of the bed slightly raised; bricks under the legs at the head of the bed is the simplest way of doing this.

Protruberant stomach

Patients with spinal osteoporosis often notice that their abdomens protrude as one of the first signs, and they may think that they are getting fatter. As explained, this is because of lack of room for all the contents of the abdomen as the spine shrinks. They must be counselled not to try and wear tight belts or corsets to push this back – it only makes the problem worse.

Sometimes they cannot eat a whole meal in comfort. Eating small meals more often helps get around this.

Stress incontinence

Patients with osteoporosis may have less control over their bladders because of the pressure in the abdomen. They may be reluctant to disclose this unless directly asked. There are ways of helping pelvic floor weakness, as it is called, and of controlling stress incontinence. Exercises to tighten up the muscles are needed.

Neck pain

Another consequence of spinal osteoporosis is the strain on the neck muscles, trying to keep the head up even though the back is bent forwards. This may require physiotherapy and special pillows on the bed at night. A neck pillow fills in the space behind the neck and allows comfortable sleep, and is available from shops or by mail order. It may be cylindrical or 'dog-bone' shaped. Some are available that are inflatable – useful in the car, chair or when you go away on holiday.

11

PRACTICAL GUIDE TO SAFETY AND COMFORT

SAFETY

If you already have established osteoporosis, in order to prevent fractures it is as important to prevent falls as it is to treat underlying bone weakness. More falls occur inside the house, in familiar surroundings, than outside the house. Although icy pavements are dangerous, most people sensibly avoid going out on them. Much more time is spent at home so there is more opportunity to fall. Hazards crop up all the time in day-to-day activities.

Sudden lifting can be dangerous. A 68-year-old woman visited her family and with joy picked up her four-year-old grandson only to get an acute pain in her back. It was so severe that she had to rest in bed for three days. She was found to have a vertebral crush fracture. If you know that you have osteoporosis, let others do the heavy lifting. One woman knew she had osteoporosis but was not going to let it bother her. She drove to the supermarket, got her shopping done, had it all put in a cardboard box at the check-out, and pushed it in a trolley to her car. Her back hurt as she tried to lift the car boot door, and became agonisingly painful as she attempted to lift the cardboard box into the boot. She drove home with great difficulty. Later the doctor arranged for an X-ray, which showed a new crush fracture of the spine.

Trivial everyday stresses can break weakened bones. A woman with osteoporosis suffered three separate episodes of rib fracture, when given a hug by her husband and loving relatives. In fact this was the way she found out that she had osteoporosis.

It is a good idea to be extra cautious when you are in a new or strange place. While staying with her son, a 60-year-old woman went to the toilet during the night. The hall was dimly lit and she did not notice her grandson's rocking horse until it was too late. She managed to put out her arm to protect herself but fractured the wrist. Even in ordinary everyday surroundings, try to take your time and look out for potential hazards. A 70-year-old woman went on holiday and on her return was met by her family. She rushed out of the station when she saw their car, did not see the kerb and fell to the ground. She could not get up and had severe pain in her hip. She had broken the proximal femur.

It is important to correct your vision and always wear the right glasses. A 63-year-old woman was tired of always having to carry around two pairs of glasses, so she got herself some bifocals. Coming downstairs in them, she looked down through the lower part of the lens meant for reading, missed her footing, fell and broke her shoulder.

Beware of the effects of any new treatments for other complaints. A 70-year-old man recently found out he had high blood pressure. One morning, shortly after his GP had prescribed a course of treatment, he got out of bed, suddenly became dizzy, fell and broke his hip. Ask whoever is prescribing your treatment about any possible problems.

CLOTHING

A high-necked dress is often uncomfortable when worn by someone whose back is rounded. Loose-fitting clothes are more comfortable. Avoid corsets. Getting a jacket or suit to fit and hang well is difficult.

Slip-on shoes or elastic laces will save having to stoop, and a dressing stick can be an invaluable aid. It is simply a stick about 12 inches (30 cm) long with a rubber grip on one end and a hook on the other that helps you get clothes on or off.

FURNITURE

Bedding
A firm mattress is important but do not trust the description 'orthopaedic' – it is often just a sales gimmick and a reason for

The following table gives a check list of ways to avoid falls.

Problem	Advice
You have already or nearly fallen because: • your knee gave way • your walking is unsteady • you were jostled by a crowd • you missed the kerb	You should use a stick, umbrella or other walking aid. In the house have solid furniture or railings on the wall to hold on to.
• you slipped on wet or icy pavements	Have shoes with a non-slip sole. Ensure the foot rubber of your walking stick is not worn.
• your vision is poor	Wear correct glasses, beware of bifocals. Have bright lighting – 'long-life' bulbs are available, which use very little electricity and can be left permanently on.
Hazards in the house: • loose rug or carpet edges; loose and trailing electrical or telephone wires	Good lighting. Tack down carpet edges and tape down loose wires.
• awkward steps in the house	Consider installing ramps and grab rails.
• children's toys left where you walk	Warn parents to keep toys off the floor – especially corridors and stairs.
• going from bed to WC at night	Fit safety lights that are left permanently on.
• in bath or shower room	Get non-skid mats and fit grab rails.
You live alone. You might not manage to get up without help if you fall.	Get a personal alarm system, linked to telephone. Get neighbours to watch out that milk and papers have been taken in.

overcharging for a hard bed. Beds which are too hard do not easily accommodate the altered shape of your spine. Try it out in the shop first. The expense of pocket-springing may be worthwhile in providing the combination of firmness and moulding to your shape. Lightweight duvets make bedmaking easier without your stooping.

Chairs and other seating

Firm upholstery with a high back to give support to the whole spine is important. They should also support the thighs and be high enough so that it is easy to get up. Several manufacturers now make suitable chairs.

It is important to rest when you can. A high stool may be useful in the kitchen and a shooting stick or fold-up chair is handy to take with you for walks so that you can have a rest wherever you are. These can be found in country sport shops.

Kitchen

A high stool is important to let you rest whilst you work, but the design of the kitchen is also important. Avoid high or deep cupboards. Use swing-out baskets that can be fitted into kitchen cupboards. Built-in appliances at working level, such as the cooker or refrigerator, are best. Microwave ovens are also helpful; they are at working level and you do not need heavy pots and pans.

You can always get advice concerning any of these ways of getting around the activities of everyday life from an occupation therapist based either in the hospital or with the social services. In some areas in the United Kingdom there are disabled living centres where you can go and look at and try some of the aids and devices that are available.

ACTIVITIES

Washing

A shower cabinet is a simple solution, and seats can often be fitted into them. If not, a bath seat helps greatly, along with a long-handled brush or sponge to get to those inaccessible parts.

Cleaning

Long handles again are a way of coping with chores such as sweeping. Long-handled dustpans and brushes are available. Find a lightweight vacuum cleaner; there are now some neat rechargeable ones available.

Driving

Use a back cushion and a secured seat-raise to make the driving position comfortable. Remember to have a head restraint to protect your neck should you stop suddenly. Adapt the seat belt so that it does not cut across your neck; several gadgets are now available for this.

COUNSELLING

As with any long-term treatment, proper counselling is essential and doctors and nurses should set aside time for this because many women conceal their worries unless encouraged to reveal them. Some women on HRT, for example, fear that the return of their periods might make pregnancy possible. It cannot, of course. And worries about cancer need to be discussed. Do not be afraid to ask your doctor about your worries.

With the current popularity of 'unorthodox', 'alternative' and 'complementary' treatments and systems of management, much misinformation – one might even say disinformation – is available on public bookshelves and in periodicals, and this may need to be discussed.

EXERCISE AND PHYSIOTHERAPY

Walking and swimming are exercises to be encouraged. Even cycling, but take care not to fall off – an exercise bike may be safer.

More specific exercises are of use to keep your spine and joints mobile, your muscles strong, your balance steady and your spine as straight as possible. Although the bones have collapsed causing the stoop, the spinal muscles can help overcome some of this. Try and stretch your arms above your head and straighten up your neck and back to make yourself as tall as possible. Do this two or three times in the morning and evening.

Manipulation by an osteopath or chiropractor, which is often used to treat ordinary back pain, is not safe in osteoporosis as the sudden movement could cause further fractures, even though it might relieve some of the old pain.

Exercises of the pelvic-floor muscles are important to prevent stress incontinence – they are the same as those that are taught to women after childbirth, and involve tensing and relaxing the muscles of the pelvic floor.

SELF-HELP SOCIETIES

In many countries self-help societies have been set up for patients with osteoporosis. In Britain there is the:

- National Osteoporosis Society
  Barton Meade House
  PO Box 10
  Radstock
  Bath BA3 3YE

This society publishes a regular newsletter where shared concerns can be aired, and much information of value to osteoporosis sufferers has already been obtained which would not normally come out in a visit to your doctor.

If we have not mentioned something in this book, then the society is sure to be able to help with your question. Where, for example, can you go to get clothes that fit your spine if it has changed shape? How can your car be adapted so that you can drive it more easily? Are there any problems with insurance or obtaining mortgages related to osteoporosis? Should you declare osteoporosis as a disability in applying for a driving licence or an insurance policy? Where can people who have difficulty seeing forwards obtain glasses with prism lenses which will enable them to see forwards even if they cannot get their heads up?

DOING EVERYTHING THAT IS NECESSARY

It must be emphasised that treatment for osteoporosis will probably never come out of a single injection or bottle of tablets. It will almost always be necessary to do all the things that are helpful. This means a good diet, plenty of calcium and exercise and, where indicated, hormone replacement therapy, calcitonin, fluoride or anabolic steroids. As the problems, such as loss of height, are not reversible, it also means attention to all those other things which follow osteoporosis and make life even more miserable.

With such attention many patients have been very considerably helped to lead a normal life, to stop having further fractures, to be able to drive and get about and not get too tired or get too much pain.

12

EXERCISE PROGRAMMES

The following chapter outlines two different exercise programmes: one for those people most at risk of osteoporosis and who are still reasonably fit and mobile; and one for those people who have already developed spinal osteoporosis.

FOR THOSE MOST AT RISK OF OSTEOPOROSIS

A daily exercise programme should consist of:
1. a 5–10 minute warm-up session to include stretching and breathing exercises;
2. followed by 20–30 minutes of general exercises, to include walking, jogging and dance orientated exercises;
3. at least 30 minutes of hard walking per day, on rough ground, slopes and stairs.

Warm up
Exercise 1. Slowly stretch your hands towards ceiling, and then towards the floor. 10 times.

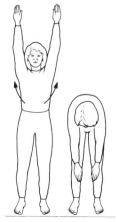

Exercise 2. With your arms straight, touch your palms together in front of you, then swing your hands out and behind you, keeping your arms at shoulder level and your palms facing backwards. 10 times

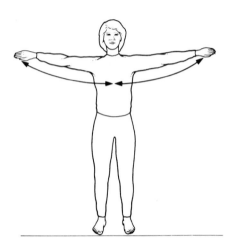

Exercise 3. 'Walk' your hands up a wall, as far as you can stretch and down again. Relax. 10 times.

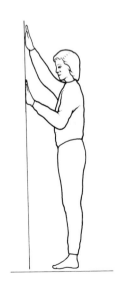

Exercise 4. With your feet shoulder-width apart, lunge sideways onto your right foot, keeping your toes facing forwards and your feet flat; sway back to the middle and then over to the left. Repeat this five times then move your feet slightly further apart and repeat the lunge from right to left a further five times.

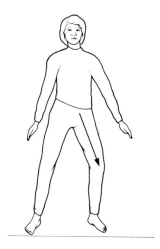

Exercise 5. With your right foot forwards, lunge your body weight forwards over your right foot. Lean your hands onto to your right knee and try to keep the toes of your right foot facing forwards. 10 times. Repeat with your left foot forward.

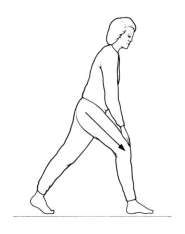

Exercise 6. With your hands on the lower part of your rib cage, breathe in deeply through your nose, feeling your rib cage expand under your hands. Hold for the count of three and then breathe out through your mouth and gently squeeze inwards with your hands. Five times.

Exercise 7. Hold onto the back of a chair, rise up on to your toes then down on to your heels and lift your toes off the floor. 20 times.

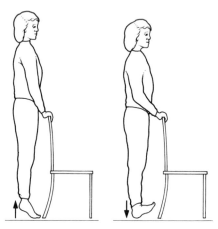

Exercise 8. Check your posture by standing with your back against a wall or a door. Keep your heels, your knees, your hips, your shoulders and the back of your head against the wall

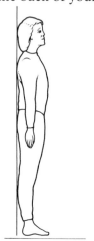

106

at all times. Walk away from the wall a few paces and maintain your upright posture, then return again to the wall and again check your posture. Three times.

Exercise 9.   Keep your arm straight, circle your right arm over your head and behind you, following with your left arm, i.e. 'back stroke'. 20 times.

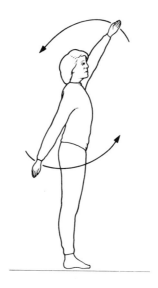

Exercise programme
Remember *never* to overtire yourself. The performance of the exercises in this session must depend on the individual's fitness.

Exercise 10.   Jog/walk on the spot for one minute.

Exercise 11. With your feet shoulder-width apart, and hands by your sides, slide your right hand down the outside of your right leg towards your foot. Stand up straight and then slide your left hand down the outside of your left leg. 10 times each side.

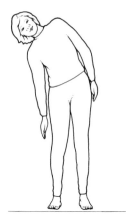

Exercise 12. With your hands on your hips and your feet apart, circle your hips to the left, to the front to the right and to the back. Repeat 10 times clockwise and 10 times anti-clockwise.

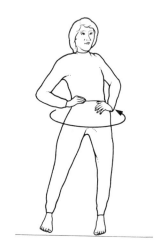

Exercise 13. Holding onto the back of a chair, bend both knees and squat down as far as you can. Stand up and straighten your legs. 10 times.

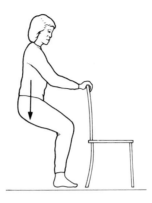

Exercise 14. Punch alternate hands towards the ceiling 10 times each hand: punch alternate hands from side to side at shoulder level 10 times each hand; punch alternate hands to the floor 10 times each hand.

Exercise 15. Side step around the room; if possible speed this up into a 'side step jog'. If you are able to, incease the width of your side step, and stretch your feet further apart.

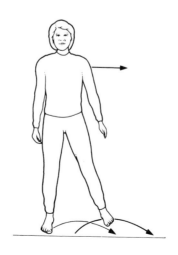

Exercise 16.   Stand with your back to a wall or a door. Place your hands, palms down, against the wall, push your hips away from the wall using your hands, arch your back and extend your head and look up towards the ceiling. Relax. 10 times.

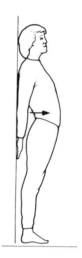

Exercise 17.   With your hands on your hips and feet apart, twist as far round to the right as you can, keeping your feet flat on the floor. Then twist round to the left as far as you can. 10 times to each side.

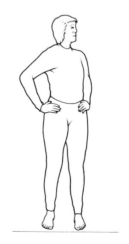

Exercise 18. Jump your feet apart and together, gradually increasing the distance between your feet. If you find this easy, jump your feet apart and then together, crossing your right leg in front of your left; then jump your feet apart and together again, crossing your left leg in front of your right. Be careful not to trip over.

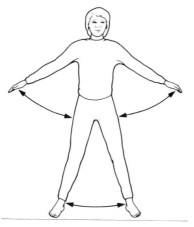

Exercise 19. Sit on a straightbacked, hard chair and fold your arms across your chest. Go from sitting to standing without using your arms, then from standing to sitting. 10 times.

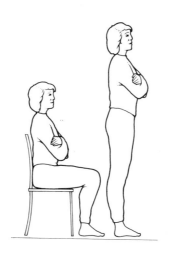

Exercise 20.   Use the bottom step of a flight of stairs. Do step-ups; lead with your right foot 10 times and then with your left foot 10 times.

Exercise 21.   Hook your fingers under a windowsill or table edge and try to 'lift' it using only your fingers. Hold for the count of 3 and relax. 10 times.

Exercise 22.   Do press-ups against a wall, hands flat, feet slightly away from the base of the wall. Bend your elbows and lower your body towards the wall, then straighten your arms and push away from the wall. If you find this easy move your feet further away from the base of the wall. 20 times.

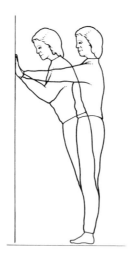

Exercise 23.   Stand sideways on to the back of a chair and hold on with the closest hand. Swing your outside leg forwards and backwards, keeping your leg as straight as possible. 10 times. Repeat with your opposite leg.

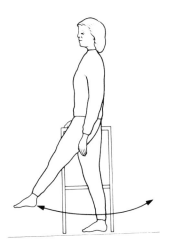

Exercise 24.   Stand sideways on to the back of a chair as above. Swing your outside leg across your supporting leg towards the chair, then swing your outside leg out and away from the chair. 10 times. Repeat with your opposite leg.

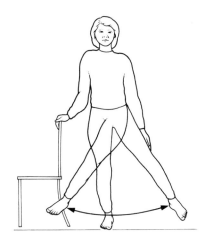

FOR THOSE WHO ALREADY HAVE SPINAL OSTEOPOROSIS

General advice

1. Exercise daily – ideally 2 short sessions per day, each lasting approximately 20 minutes.
2. Go for daily walks, for pleasure if not for a purpose, e.g. to the shops, only not when you are anticipating lots of shopping to carry.
3. Take care how you lift even the lightest of loads. Use your leg muscles, it is what they were designed for.
4. Do not forget that exercise is important, not only for your bones but also your heart, lungs, circulation, muscles and joints.
5. Enjoy exercising! Choose an appropriate time when you are unlikely to be disturbed; exercise to your favourite music; vary your routine by setting yourself a set number of repetitions per exercise or count the number of repetitions per exercise in one minute – the choice is endless!

Those people who already have spinal osteoporosis should pay special attention to:

Posture. Perform regular, daily postural checks and exercises. Check your posture against a wall; correct your posture in front of a mirror.

Relief of muscle spasm and tension. Use relaxation techniques, hot baths, heat lamps, massage.

Breathing exercises. These are vitally important to maintain the mobility of your rib cage and your lungs.

Muscle strength –
- *postural muscles.* ie legs, back, abdominals.
- *shoulder girdle muscles, arms and neck*
- *pelvic floor muscles*, the muscles which help to give you voluntary control over your bladder and your bowel, and control the urge to pass water or to stop the flow of water midstream. The easiest way to exercise these muscles is to lie on your back with your knees bent and your feet flat on

114

the bed/floor. Place your hands on your stomach, now tighten your stomach muscles, tighten the muscles between your legs and tighten your buttock muscles together at the same time. It should feel as though you are 'pulling-up' inside you. Hold for the count of 3 and relax.

Warm up
Try the stretching and breathing exercises in the warm-up session of the exercise programme for those at risk.

Exercise Programme

Standing

Exercise 1.   Arms above head, stretch lower. Breathe in as you raise your arms and breathe out as you lower your arms. 10 times. (See Exercise 1 in the 'risk' programme.)

Exercise 2.   Do side bends, left and right. 10 times each side. (See Exercise 11 in the 'risk' programme.)

Exercise 3.   Slump forwards and down, then stand up straight and arch back.

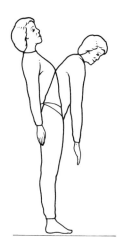

Exercise 4. Swing one arm up and back, the other down and back, swing and change. 10 times.

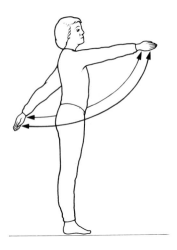

Exercise 5. With your hands on your shoulders, touch your elbows in front of your chest then push your elbows out behind you. 10 times.

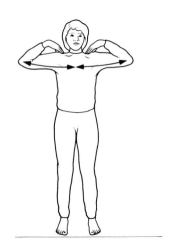

Sitting

Exercise 6. Slump forwards, hands on hips, sit up straight then arch backwards. 10 times.

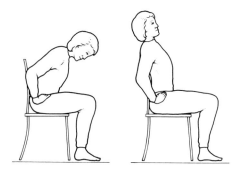

Exercise 7. With your hands on your hips, and feet flat on the floor, twist to the right and then to the left. 10 times.

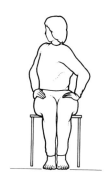

Exercise 8. Straighten your right leg out in front of you, then your left. 10 times each leg.

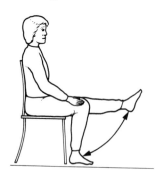

Lying

Exercise 9. With your knees bent, arch the small of your back away from the bed, then press the small of your back down. 10 times.

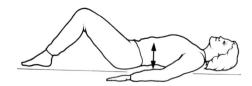

Exercise 10. Raise your hips off the bed as high as you can and arch your back. 10 times.

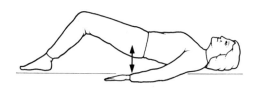

Exercise 11. Roll both knees from side to side. 10 times each side.

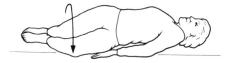

Exercise 12. Brace your knees down into the bed and relax. 10 times.

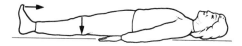

Exercise 13. Put your hands on the fronts of your thighs, then stretch both arms right above your head, towards the floor behind you and rest. 10 times.

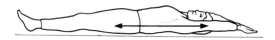

Exercise 14. Stretch your hands towards the ceiling, then lower your hands to the floor at your shoulder level, and lift up again. 5 times.

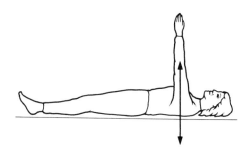

Exercise 15.   Put your hands on your lower ribs on each side, breathe slowly and gently in through your nose as deeply as you can, then breathe out through your mouth and gently squeeze inwards with your hands.

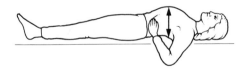

Note.   It is very important to check your posture *every day* – an easy way to do this is to stand with your back against a wall or a door, with your heels, your knees, your hips, your shoulders and the *back* of your head against the door!

Neck exercises

Sit in a comfortable chair, ideally with your head and shoulders supported. Do these exercises slowly and gently to avoid sharp muscle jerks or dizziness.

Exercise 16.   Bend your right ear down towards your right shoulder. Do not let your right shoulder creep up towards your ear. Rest and repeat to your left. Five times to each side.

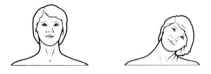

Exercise 17.   Turn to look over your right shoulder, keeping your body steady and your chin parallel to the floor. Repeat to the left. 5 times to each side.

Exercise 18. Keeping your chin parallel to the floor, retract your chin backwards on to your shoulders, give yourself as many double chins as possible. 5 times.

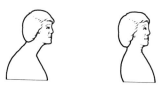

Exercise 19. Chin to your chest as far as you can, now tip your head backwards and look towards the ceiling. SLOWLY 5 times.

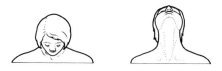

Prone lying, i.e. flat on your front

Only attempt these exercises if you feel happy in this position and are able to get yourself into and out of the position.

Exercise 20. With your arms straight, lift both hands off the floor as high as you can; if possible lift your head and shoulders as well. Hold, then lower. 10 times.

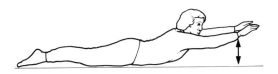

Exercise 21.   Bend both knees, heels as close to your bottom as you can, lift your thighs off the bed, if possible. Hold and lower. 10 times.

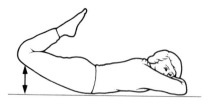

Exercise 22.   Legs straight, lift alternate legs on the bed, keeping your leg as straight as possible.

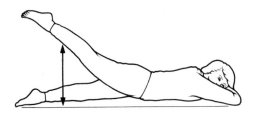

13

OTHER DISEASES WHICH CAUSE BONE PAIN OR FRACTURE

Other diseases which cause bone pain or fractures and which might be confused with osteoporosis include:
- Diseases which cause general loss of bone density.
- Diseases which cause shortening of the spine and a bent back.
- Conditions which cause local changes in bone.

GENERAL LOSS OF BONE DENSITY

Myelomatosis
This is a cancer of the bone marrow or, more specifically, of the 'plasma cells' in the bone marrow responsible for making antibodies against invading micro-organisms. This cancer spreads within the bone and produces a kind of rogue antibody in vast quantities, at the expense of normal antibodies. The diagnosis is made by detecting this rogue antibody in the blood or in the urine.

The resemblance to osteoporosis can be close, including wedging and collapse of the vertebrae, with loss of height and rounding of the back. It can be distinguished from osteoporosis by readily available tests. Treatment with anti-cancer drugs can prolong life and relieve pain, but a complete cure is unlikely.

Osteomalacia
Osteomalacia or 'adult rickets' results from depletion of the body stores of vitamin D.

If you put a bone in a weak acid, it will not change shape, but it will become soft enough to be cut easily with a knife. What you have done is dissolve out the bone mineral but leave the bone matrix, the scaffolding of fibres and other substances, on which the bone mineral crystals are deposited.

In life, when bone is continuously being dissolved and continuously being replaced, the replacement is begun by first forming more bone matrix. Almost immediately the mineral is added, a process requiring the presence of vitamin D. So if there is inadequate vitamin D, the matrix accumulates and can very easily be seen under the microscope. Naturally, bone which is not properly mineralised is weak and may develop painful local cracks or may fracture right through. This is osteomalacia. It can and often does exist as a mixed bone disease with osteoporosis.

Lack of both sunlight and dietary vitamin D will cause osteomalacia. So will conditions such as gastrectomy (removal of the stomach) which causes malabsorption of vitamin D, or liver or kidney conditions which interfere with the conversion of vitamin D into the final active product.

Osteomalacia in adults (and rickets in children) used to be common in the past, particularly in the north of England and the industrial towns of Scotland, due to a combination of little exposure to sunlight and a poor diet. It is now largely confined to Asian women living in these areas whose custom is not to expose their skins when out of doors, or to the elderly who do not go out much and live behind glass (ordinary window glass does not allow the vitamin D-forming ultraviolet rays in sunlight to reach them).

Osteomalacia is cured in most cases by restoring vitamin D, either as sunlight's effect on the skin or in the diet. Many foods contain vitamin D; it is added in small quantities to margarines and to breakfast cereals, for example. The commonest natural food source is fish, especially oily fish such as herrings, mackerel and salmon.

There are many forms of vitamin D and labelling of these in manufactured foods can be confusing, so they are best described by their activity in terms of international units, not by weight – 400 international units is the daily requirement for an adult. More than this is unnecessary, and much more (as can be obtained in halibut liver oil preparations) can be harmful. And vitamin D in very large doses has been used as a rat poison!

Hyperparathyroidism

This is what happens when there is an overproduction of parathyroid hormone by the parathyroid glands, four little glands which lie in the neck. Their job is to regulate the level of calcium dissolved in the bloodstream. When they are overactive the blood level of calcium rises too high. The kidneys try to correct this by excreting more calcium and phosphate in the urine, and this loss of calcium in the urine has to be made up by dissolving more from the bones. Hyperparathyroidism, if severe, is treated by surgical operation.

Hyperparathyroidism differs from osteoporosis in that the levels of calcium in the blood are high, not low. This makes the sufferer feel ill, and pass a lot of urine. The brain may be affected, so sufferers get depressed and have psychological problems. The drain of calcium out of the bones into the urine means that many sufferers develop kidney stones.

Osteogenesis imperfecta

This is a rare disease of special interest to this book. It is true 'brittle-bone disease', although that name is often applied to osteoporosis. It is a rare inherited disorder of the collagen fibres which give strength to normal bone.

Very severe forms of osteogenesis imperfecta are not compatible with life because the bones are so brittle that all the ribs and spine collapse. However, children with milder forms of brittle-bone disease suffer many fractures during normal play. This can be doubly distressing to the parents, who can find themselves accused of baby battering. The tendency to fracture gets less if the child survives to adolescence, but in girls it may return again at the time of the menopause. Such late examples of mild brittle-bone disease cannot easily be distinguished from ordinary osteoporosis except by the characteristic changes in other members of the family.

DISEASES WHICH CAUSE A BENT BACK

Senile kyphosis

In senile kyphosis (curved spine in old age) the shoulders are rounded, the back behind the chest is curved forward, and the head has to be held up hard by the neck muscles in order to see forwards. There is a loss of height. It can in fact look very like spinal osteoporosis.

But this is not caused by collapsing bones. It is caused by shrinkage and drying up of the intervertebral discs, the rubbery structures which lie between the bones of the spine.

Adolescent kyphosis

Scheuerman's disease or adolescent kyphosis is a disorder of the growth of the spine seen in adolescent boys and young men who develop a permanently rounded back. When they are old men this may at first sight look like osteoporosis, but the appearance on X-ray is different.

Ankylosing spondylitis

Ankylosing spondylitis (or 'poker back' disease) is a rheumatic disease, a painful form of arthritis of the spine. Young men are affected more often than young women. In bad cases the spine becomes rigid (ankylosed), a solid rod of bone. When this happens there is no movement and so no pain. Untreated or badly treated sufferers get set in the sort of position they would have sitting at a low table or driving a car – when they stand up they have the shape of a question mark.

WEDGING AND COLLAPSE OF VERTEBRAE

The commonest cause of wedging or collapse of vertebrae is probably trauma – a road traffic accident, a fall from a horse, a fall on the stairs landing heavily on the buttocks are all common causes. One vertebra may 'give' painfully. Often this is not discovered until years later when the person is X-rayed for some other cause. A wedged vertebra caused by trauma is harmless once it is healed, and it will not interfere with life.

Much more serious is the spread of cancer to the spine. The cancer is usually from the breast in women, the prostate in men or from the lungs in smokers. Modern treatments can do a great deal to relieve pain and restore health in breast and prostate cancer, but very little can be done for spinal cancer that has spread from the lung. This sort of cancer can usually be found to be the cause of the wedged vertebrae by a full examination by a doctor and some further X-rays and blood tests.

Infections of the vertebrae occur and may also cause spinal collapse. At one time this was almost always due to tuberculosis and was called Pott's disease. It affected children and adolescents and they would grow up with terrible hunched backs. Today infections by other micro-organisms are more common. It is a serious condition, dangerous to life, and requires prompt treatment with antibiotics.

DISEASES WHICH CAUSE LOCAL CHANGES IN BONES AND JOINTS

Neck and back pain
Neck and back pain is increasingly common as one gets older. Osteoporosis may cause this, but more frequently it is the result of thinning and stiffness of the intervertebral discs in the neck and spine. This causes strains in the spinal joints and sometimes trapping of the nerves as they leave the spine, causing pain, 'pins and needles' and even numbness in the arms or legs.

Easily broken limbs
Easily broken limb bones are not always caused by osteoporosis. A typical story might be that a woman goes out for a walk and some shopping. Whilst walking one leg breaks in the thigh and she falls to the ground. This is called a pathological fracture and is often the result of the spread of a cancer into the bone. The X-rays of the broken bone usually reveal this to be the cause, and the original site of the cancer is discovered by a full examination and further tests. Cancer of the breast in women, the prostate in men and the lung in smokers are the usual causes. Surgeons often put a steel rod through the hollow bone bridging the gap where the cancer has attacked it. This makes walking possible again.

Paget's disease
Paget's disease of the bone is a curious condition in which virus-like particles appear in certain bones. These particles look very like measles virus or dog distemper virus, but are not the same. The cells in affected bones become very active, both in dissolving bone mineral and in building it up again. Very often the whole process is painless and only discovered

in a chance X-ray. But in some the balance between demineralising and remineralising is upset, so the affected bone (or bones, because sometimes several bones are involved) becomes either osteoporotic or very dense. The bones may change shape and, when thinned, they may break.

Very active Paget's disease is associated with a large increase in the blood supply to the bone, so that if the shin bone is involved it feels hot to the touch. Paget's disease of this sort can be painful, especially at night. It can also cause pain if the disease gets into the bones of a joint, causing them to change shape and no longer fit each other properly. Or it can be painful because of cracks or even complete fractures. If it affects a bone in the spine it may compress nerves coming from the spine, and if the skull is affected the sufferer becomes deaf because bone overgrowth compresses the sensitive internal ear.

Fortunately the condition can be suppressed and pain (if due directly to the condition) relieved rapidly by calcitonin. Bisphosphonates (diphosphonates) and mythramycin are other useful drugs for Paget's disease.

LOCAL OSTEOPOROSIS

Any disused limb will lose bone density, whether the disuse is the result of paralysis, immobilisation, for example in plaster after a fracture, or because of pain on movement. So painful arthritis confined to one knee will be followed by local osteoporosis in that leg. Poliomyelitis (infantile paralysis) always causes osteoporosis in the paralysed limb.

There are also some rare but unpleasant conditions called Sudek's atrophy or algodystrophy where not only the bone but the overlying skin and flesh waste away painfully. There is no good treatment but in many patients the condition recovers in time.

14

SUFFERERS' QUESTIONS AND ANSWERS

DIET

• Are special diets/slimming diets harmful or helpful?

Body fat has some advantages. Following the menopause it makes small but important amounts of oestrogens which help protect the skeleton. So one should not be too thin. It is important to take sufficient calcium and trace amounts of fluoride in the diet, but too much protein may be harmful, and too much bran will stop you absorbing all the calcium from the food that you eat.

• Do I need vitamin pills?

A good balanced diet should give adequate vitamins. The vitamin that is most important for bone is vitamin D, and this is mainly made in the skin by the action of sunlight. It is also found in fish oil, but only a small amount is needed as too much may be harmful.

• Do remedies such as cod liver oil, evening primrose oil or green lipped muscle extract help?

Cod liver oil is a useful source of vitamin D, but only a small amount of this is needed. There is no evidence to suggest evening primrose oil or green lipped muscle helps osteoporosis.

• I eat all the right things and keep to a fat-free diet.

You may eat all the right things, but a fat-free diet may be low in calcium.

- I have gallstones and I am on a very restricted fat-free diet.

Skimmed milk contains plenty of calcium and minimal fat.

- I have always eaten a well balanced diet – fresh fruit, vegetables and not too much red meat or dairy products – but now I am told that my spine has collapsed because of osteoporosis. Why?

For some reason red meat and dairy products have become the root of all evil. The lack of dairy products may mean that you have taken too little calcium in your diet.

- I have been taking lots of dairy products but I was told by doctors that it does not make any difference and that it is not good for my heart.

Calcium is important and dairy products are the best source. Skimmed milk avoids the problems with the heart. But calcium supplements cannot cure the deficiency of female sex hormones which occurs after the menopause.

- I am a 39-year-old female and a vegan, which means that I do not eat animal flesh and dairy products. I am very active in sports like swimming and hill walking. I eat plenty of beans, pulses, wholemeal rice and flours. What particular foods should I eat to increase my calcium intake and help prevent me from developing osteoporosis?

Green vegetables contain calcium but the roughage in the other foods you eat much of will hinder its absorption. It may be necessary for you to use calcium tablets to supplement your diet.

TREATMENT

- The doctor has given me painkillers which I do not like to keep taking as I live alone and am worried that they may make me ill or I may become dependent on them.

Painkillers such as paracetamol can be very effective, have very few side effects and you do not become dependent on them.

- I have taken calcium tablets but they have not helped the pain in my back.

Calcium tablets will not relieve the pain in the back. They are given to prevent further loss of bone and fractures.

- I suffer from serious back pains and my doctor says this is because I lack calcium in my bones and they are weak. I am taking calcium tablets to strengthen my bones. Will this help?

Yes, but it will be more effective with hormone replacement therapy.

- I am 44 years old and seven years ago I was diagnosed as having osteoporosis. Since then I have been treated with hormone replacement, calcium and a small amount of vitamin D. I still however get a lot more pain than I feel I should get with being on all this replacement therapy. Why is this treatment not working?

The treatment is to prevent worsening of the osteoporosis and unfortunately does not always relieve all the pain. The way of seeing if this is working is whether the loss of bone is reduced and fractures prevented.

- I am now 64 years old and my doctor has just diagnosed osteoporosis of my spine. Needless to say, my male doctor at the time of my menopause did not agree with hormone replacement therapy. Am I now too old to benefit from this treatment?

Some gynaecologists say that no woman is too old to benefit from HRT. It will not put bone back but will prevent further loss, and if one is prepared to put up with the return of periods then it is worth considering.

- I am 58 years old and have osteoporosis of the spine. I have continuous back pain and have found no benefit from osteopaths, chiropracters or from acupuncture.

Back pain may be caused by muscle spasm and this sometimes improves with acupuncture, but manipulation of a fragile spine is not without risk.

131

- Is it true that after the menopause a woman cannot absorb sufficient extra calcium, so it is no good altering one's diet to take more calcium.

The gut is less efficient at absorbing calcium as you get older, but if you take more in the diet then sufficient will be absorbed by the body.

- I had my menopause four years ago and I have been advised by one doctor to have a hysterectomy and take HRT, and by another to just take calcium tablets.

Hormone replacement therapy is the most effective way of preventing osteoporosis following the menopause. Following a hysterectomy oestrogen alone can be used and this will not only prevent osteoporosis but will reduce the risk of ischaemic heart disease. HRT can be given quite safely in the presence of the womb if a progestogen is given for 10–12 days each cycle. Calcium is not as effective as hormones, but a lower dose of HRT is effective if plenty of calcium is taken at the same time.

- My periods are beginning to become irregular so I persuaded my doctor to start HRT. I unfortunately suffered discomfort and pain in my breasts and nipples during the second half of each cycle so that I could not continue. I also had recurrence of periods, which were painful and heavy. I have not been able to continue with HRT because of this.

Some people suffer such problems with HRT. Sometimes these can be avoided by trying different preparations. A lower dose may be tolerated and this would be effective in preventing osteoporosis if plenty of calcium is taken at the same time.

- I have cancer of the breast and have had radiotherapy to my ovaries. I am worried that I may develop osteoporosis.

Unfortunately cancer of the breast is one reason for not taking HRT. As you have had radiotherapy to your ovaries it may be that the cancer grows in the presence of sex hormones and it is therefore unadvisable to take them. It is worthwhile taking plenty of calcium and exercise in an attempt to prevent osteoporosis. Calcitonin injections might be used in a specialised clinic.

ESTABLISHED OSTEOPOROSIS

- Thirty years ago I had a hysterectomy and removal of both my ovaries. I had an oestrogen implant immediately following the operation but no further hormone therapy has been given. Seven years ago I fell down a few steps and sustained multiple fractures of my tibia and fibula. I now also have back pain and X-rays have shown thinning of the bones, with two collapsed vertebrae.

The removal of the ovaries before the natural menopause will almost certainly have caused osteoporosis and you did not have HRT for long enough to prevent it. Once the bones are thinned and weak they will break more easily.

- I have started getting pain in my back and have lost 2 inches in height. Bending over an upright hoover, cleaning and gardening have become extremely painful. I am 75 years old. Two spinal bones gave way three years ago. They initially hurt but after resting for a week they have been no trouble. Last year another vertebra painfully collapsed but the pain went after a few weeks. I have shrunk from 5 foot to 4 foot 7 inches. The curving worsens my hiatus hernia and now my stomach sticks out.

Unfortunately these are the typical problems of osteoporosis, but we have discovered ways of overcoming some of these problems (see Chapters 10 and 11).

- A precautionary X-ray last year after pulling some muscles badly in my lower back revealed that my bones were thin and one of my lumbar vertebrae was partially collapsed. I get problems with standing and walking and I am only pain free if I sit or lie down. I am 63 years.

Collapse of a vertebra can follow very minor trauma, such as just pulling a muscle. It is important to strengthen your spinal muscles and improve your posture (see suggested exercise programme on page 103).

- I am a sufferer of osteoporosis, having a curved spine and loss of height. I was only 5 foot but I am now 4 foot 10 inches. I shall be 68 next month. I am now finding it difficult to do the housework.

The daily chores in the house can be helped by using various aids (see Chapter 11). You should seek the advice of an occupational therapist.

- I am 74, and 12 years ago I noticed that I could no longer reach up to close the window. I was shrinking and becoming stooped. I am now only 4 foot 7 inches; clothes no longer fit me and they cut into my neck. I cannot get through to the doctor – he does not seem to understand what I mean.

Osteoporosis has long been considered just a natural part of getting old. Doctors are now becoming increasingly aware of the problems of the osteoporotic sufferer. If you are unhappy with your own doctor, you can always change.

- I have osteoporosis. I was manually cleaning a big carpet and pulling it across the room to dry when I developed back pain. They gave me a surgical corset which was very uncomfortable and after a while I could not bear to wear it.

Surgical corsets are not very helpful in osteoporosis. It is usually the upper spine that is affected, but the corset mainly supports the lower spine. They squash the protruding stomach and are uncomfortable.

- I have shrunk from 5 foot 10 inches down to 5 foot in two years and I have lost five vertebrae. Why is this, and what can I do to prevent this worsening?

You clearly have marked osteoporosis. Your doctor may consider HRT and fluoride to prevent it worsening if this can be properly supervised locally.

- How much should I do? How far should I walk?

The more active you can keep the better, but this should not be at the expense of causing a lot of pain. It is a matter of finding your exercise tolerance. Walking a few miles a week will help protect the skeleton.

- I was put on steroids 15 years ago for a serious chest problem when I was 32 and this has caused osteoporosis. I have broken ribs on several occasions, just from bending down, and I am always very frightened when the winter comes, with ice and snow, in case I fall. The pain is the worst problem. Tablets are of little help but a course of acupuncture helped a lot.

Steroids if taken for many years do cause osteoporosis. Acupuncture will not prevent or cure this, but may be helpful in relieving the pain from it.

- I have osteoporosis. Some days I can hardly walk because of the constant pain in my back. I spend nights in the chair because I can no longer bear to lie on the bed. I take painkillers but they do not help much. I am 75 years old.

The treatments for osteoporosis such as HRT and calcium do not relieve the pain but prevent further bone loss and fracture. It is a matter of finding painkillers which help, or using other methods of pain relief such as electrical stimulation (TENS). Improving posture with exercises may also help.

SYMPTOMS NOT DUE TO OSTEOPOROSIS

- I am concerned about the persistent weakness I have in my wrists, ankles, hips and shoulders.

- Since my hysterectomy I have had pains in my joints which are getting worse. Is this osteoporosis?

- I am 57 years of age and had a hysterectomy with removal of the ovaries when I was 46. I now get pain in my neck, shoulders, back and knees. Is this due to osteoporosis?

- Three years ago I had my right ovary removed and since then I have had backache and now my left hip is beginning to hurt.

Osteoporosis does not cause weakness or pain about the joints. It does cause collapse of vertebrae, which may result in back pain and an increased risk of fracturing other bones.

- I am now 65 years old and have gradually become stooped. My doctor tells me the X-ray does not show osteoporosis but shows narrowing of the disc spaces.

Loss of height and curvature of the spine may result from thinning of the discs between the vertebrae due to disc degeneration, and this can look very much like, but is not, osteoporosis.

PREVENTION

- I am generally healthy and keep my weight to 8 stone. I am 5 foot 9 inches.

Keeping too thin may not be of benefit as body fat is important after the menopause as a source of sex hormones.

- I am 45 years old, so coming up to the menopause soon, and should like to do all I can to prevent osteoporosis if possible.

HRT is the most effective way of preventing osteoporosis, but should be taken for several years, not just months.

- I do not like taking drugs.

HRT is the most effective way of preventing osteoporosis and in a way one is using natural products that have merely been recreated in a laboratory. Calcium is a normal part of a diet, and exercise does not need a prescription.

RISK FACTORS AND SPECIFIC CAUSES

- I am 67 and never had back trouble before, but I am developing rounded shoulders. I am in so much pain and I cannot do things as I used to. I have good food, have never smoked or taken any alcohol in my life and always walked a lot. Why have I now got this problem?

Unfortunately we do not know enough about the cause of osteoporosis to pick out all those who are at risk. Even having done all the right things, some people will still suffer from the disease.

- My grandmother and her two daughters, one being my mother, had osteoporosis. I have not yet reached the menopause. What should I do?

A family history of osteoporosis does increase the risk of developing it. This has to be weighed up with other risk factors, but may be good grounds to consider HRT when you reach the menopause.

- My fingernails are extremely brittle and flake off like fish scales. Is this a forewarning of bones lacking calcium?

Fingernails are made of keratin. There is no known link with osteoporosis.

- I have been on steroids for almost 11 years after a successful renal transplant, but eight months ago fell and broke my hip. I am now 53 years old (male).

Corticosteroids are essential following renal transplantation, but unfortunately cause osteoporosis. Calcium supplements prevent some of the loss of bone that is caused by these steroids.

- About six years ago my doctor put me on steroids. I had not taken them very long when, whilst sitting in my sitting room, the door bell rang. I got up, crossed the room and suddenly went 'Oh, my back!' and collapsed. Since then I have had back pain and have been unable to go out on my own, walk with a stick and cannot stand too long.

Unfortunately, vertebrae may collapse without any trauma if they are sufficiently weakened by osteoporosis.

- My two-year-old daughter is on steroids for asthma and does not like milk.

Corticosteroids in childhood also cause osteoporosis. This effect is reduced if the dose is given on alternate days. Calcium is probably important and can be given as supplements if not taken in the diet. She may like yoghurts or cheese.

- I am concerned about osteoporosis since my menopause happened over 20 years ago, when I was 41. Should I be taking HRT?

Unfortunately you will have had 20 years of bone loss, but further loss would probably be prevented by commencing HRT now, if you are prepared to suffer periods.

- I have an 18-year-old daughter allergic to cheese and milk products. What should she do to prevent the risk of later osteoporosis?

It may be necessary to take calcium supplements to provide an adequate amount to preserve bone strength if dairy products cannot be tolerated. Ask her to try goat's milk or sheep's milk products. She may be able to take these.

- My husband had his pituitary gland removed and has to take steroids for the rest of his life. I am now worried that he will develop osteoporosis.

Because the pituitary gland has been removed the body will not make those steroids which are essential for life. The amount being given is equivalent to that which the body would have made and should not cause osteoporosis. It is only when excessive steroids are used for treatment of disease that there is a risk of osteoporosis.

- I am 47 years of age and feel well at the moment but dread the thought of ending up like my mother who has broken many bones from simple falls. Is it hereditary?

If your mother has osteoporosis, then there is an increased chance of you also developing it and it is worth considering HRT. Certainly you should take plenty of calcium and exercise.

- I suffer from Crohn's disease and am treated with corticosteroids. I cannot take much in the way of dairy products.

Calcium can be taken in other ways, and it is certainly advisable to ensure you are taking 1.5 g a day.

HORMONE REPLACEMENT THERAPY

- I am 38 years old and for the last four years have had severe menopausal symptoms after the removal of my ovaries. Am I at greater risk of osteoporosis because of this?

Yes, and you should seriously consider taking HRT.

- My own doctor does not believe in hormone replacement

therapy and there is no local menopause clinic. Where can I go to receive such treatment?

Many doctors are still concerned about the risks of HRT, but new information is showing this treatment to be safe. If you cannot persuade your doctor it may be necessary to consider changing to a different practitioner.

- I am wanting to take HRT but I am worried that I will put on weight and that there is a risk of cancer.

Weight gain is normally not great. There is no real risk of cancer with modern use of this treatment.

- I am now 45 years old but had my menopause at 39. I eat a good diet of calcium-rich foods and do a lot of exercise. I was on HRT for five years but unfortunately had to stop due to continual pre-menstrual tension.

Some hormone replacement preparations are better tolerated than others. A lower dose can be used in combination with calcium, with the same benefit.

- I have breast cancer and cannot take HRT. Is there any alternative in order to prevent osteoporosis?

Plenty of calcium and exercise. Calcitonin can be used but it means regular injections.

- I am 51 years old and have osteoporosis. I had my ovaries removed 10 years ago but I never had hormone replacement. I was told that I was too old to need it.

You were not too old to need HRT and it is not too late to start now in order to prevent the situation worsening. Even following the menopause some sex hormones come from the ovaries, and these should be replaced.

- I have osteoporosis of the spine and I am worried that HRT will increase my weight and put excessive stress on my back.

The weight gain with HRT is not great and unlikely to worsen your symptoms.

- I have had a hysterectomy and my ovaries removed and the

gynaecologist recommended oestrogen replacement. People have told me however that it causes cancer.

Oestrogen alone does increase the risk of cancer of the womb but as you have had this removed it does not pose a problem. There has been some concern that the risk of breast cancer could be increased; the information we have suggests that if there is an increased risk of breast cancer, then it is extremely small and should not dissuade you from hormone replacement therapy.

- I am 30 years old and my periods have stopped. I was shocked when my gynaecologist told me that the investigations showed that I was having an early menopause. I find the thought of taking hormone replacement therapy for the rest of my life rather daunting.

The early loss of periods is a major risk factor for developing osteoporosis and this can be prevented by hormone replacement therapy. The longer one takes hormone replacement, the longer any possibility of osteoporosis is deferred. It would be advisable in your case to take it at least up to the age of the expected menopause – about 50 years of age. Continuing to take adequate calcium in the diet and plenty of exercise is also important.

EXERCISE

I am 64 years of age and have osteoporosis of my spine. I try to exercise, but which form of exercise is best? Would a little cycling do any harm? How far should I walk?

The best exercises are those which put a stress on the limbs, but you do not want to risk falling. An exercise bicycle may be better than cycling along the road. Walking is also excellent; 5 miles a week is plenty.

- What exercises should I do to avoid the bad posture that I am developing with my osteoporosis.

A simple programme of exercises is given on page 116.

GLOSSARY

absorptiometry Also known as densitometry. Measuring the amount of radiation energy that a bone obstructs. Osteoporotic or 'thin' bones allow more radiation to pass through than do normal dense bones.

ACTH Adrenocorticotrophic hormone. One of the pituitary hormones which influence other hormone-producing glands, in this case the adrenal glands.

adrenal glands Two small hormone-producing glands that sit on top of the kidneys.

amenorrhoea Loss of menstrual periods.

anabolic steroids Synthetic hormones similar to androgens. They increase muscle bulk and muscle bone strength.

androgens Male sex hormones produced in the testes.

atrophy Wasting away.

biopsy Taking a small piece of tissue from someone for examination under the microscope. Bone biopsy is usually done near the iliac crest (part of the pelvis).

bisphosphonates Also called diphosphonates. Chemical compounds which can affect the formation and the dissolving of the crystals of bone mineral.

BMC Bone mineral content, usually expressed as the amount of calcium per unit volume of bone.

bone mass The amount of bone tissue in a bone. It consists of bone mineral (hydroxyapatite) and the framework of collagen fibres embedded in it, but not the bone marrow which occupies the hollow spaces in a bone.

calciferol One form of vitamin D.

calcitonin A hormone produced by the thyroid gland in the neck. It regulates the activity of the living bone cells and the amount of calcium in the blood.

calories   Units of energy value. A calorie is the amount of heat which will raise the temperature of 1 gram of water by one degree celsius.

Calorie   A Calorie (large C) is 1,000 calories. Used to measure the energy value of foods.

CAT scan   Computerised axial tomography scan. A type of X-ray imaging which can look at the internal structure of the body in detail. It can be adapted to measure bone mineral content.

cervix   Means the neck, so a painful neck might be diagnosed as 'cervical spondylosis'. (Also used for the neck of the womb – hence cervical smear, cervical cancer.)

climacteric   Another name for the menopause.

collagen   The tough fibres that hold the body together. Meshworks of collagen fibres give strength to the skin. Bundles of collagen fibres form tendons which attach muscles to bone, and ligaments which protect joints from hingeing in the wrong direction. Collagen fibres are also embedded in bone to give it greater strength.

compact bone   Forms the dense outer part of a bone, the cortex.

cortex   Literally means the bark of tree. Used to describe the outer part of bone, hence cortical bone. Also used to describe the outer part of the adrenal gland.

corticosteroids   Hormones produced by the adrenal cortex. One of them is cortisone.

crush fracture   A fracture of one of the bones in the spine, which is crushed rather than being snapped.

Cushing's syndrome   Caused by too much corticosteroid hormone, and leads to osteoporosis.

diphosphonate   See **bisphosphonate.**

diuretic   A drug which makes you pass more urine.

dual-photon absorptiometry   Absorptiometry using radiation of two different wavelengths. This makes it easier to distinguish bone and soft tissues than single-photon absorptiometry.

endometrium   The lining of the womb. Hence endometrial cancer.

femur   The long bone in the thigh. In osteoporosis any fracture is usually in or near the neck of the femur, near the hip joint. This is commonly known as fractured hip.

fibroid   A non-malignant tumour of the wall of the womb.

142

flat bones These comprise the pelvis, shoulder blades and the skull, and consist of a thin layer of medulla sandwiched between two layers of cortical bone.

follicle The nest of cells surrounding a developing egg in the ovary. It makes the female sex hormones oestrogen and progesterone.

FSH Follicle stimulating hormone. One of the pituitary hormones which influence other hormone-producing glands, in this case the ovaries.

g Gram. There are roughly 28 grams in an ounce.

hormone A chemical messenger, secreted by a gland in one part of the body and carried round the body in the bloodstream to influence the growth, development or activity of another part.

humerus The long bone in the upper arm. In osteoporosis it usually fractures very close to the shoulder joint.

hydroxyapatite The name for bone mineral. A compound of calcium, phosphate and water.

hyper- Too much of something.

hypo- Too little of something.

hysterectomy Removal of the womb.

idiopathic Means 'caused itself'. Used about osteoporosis when the cause is unknown.

iliac crest The part of the pelvic bone just below the waist.

intervertebral disc Cushion-like structures between the bones (vertebrae) of the spine, which allow the spine to bend.

kyphosis Increased forward curvature of the spine. A hunched back.

l Litre. Roughly 1⅔ UK pints or 2 US pints.

lactase The enzyme which breaks down milk sugar (lactose). Lactase is missing in some people, who cannot tolerate milk as a result.

LH Luteinising hormone. One of the pituitary hormones which influence other hormone-producing glands, in this case the ovaries.

long bone Tubular bones, such as the femur, humerus and finger bones. (As opposed to 'flat' bones.)

medulla The middle of a bone, where most of the bone marrow is found.

menarche The age of onset of menstruation.

menopause The last menstrual period.

mg Milligram, a thousandth of a gram, 0.001 g.

μg   Microgram, a millionth of a gram, 0.000,001 g. Some vitamins are measured in micrograms in the small-print contents label on packets of food.

ml   Millilitre, one thousandth of a litre, 0.001 l; 1 ml of water weighs 1 gram.

MRI   Magnetic resonance imaging. A method of imaging the inside of the body using tuned magnetic fields instead of X-rays. It 'sees' the wetter parts of the body rather than the drier parts, so the brain shows up more clearly than the skull, the bone marrow more clearly than the bone itself, and osteoporotic bones are clearer than healthy bones.

oestrogen   Female sex hormone, produced mainly in the ovaries.

oophorectomy   Removal of the ovaries. In salpingo-oophorectomy, the tubes leading from the ovary to the womb are also removed. Bilateral oophorectomy means that both ovaries have been removed.

osteoblast   The cells that build up bone tissue.

osteoclast   The cells that dissolve bone tissue.

osteomalacia   The bone disease caused by lack of vitamin D.

osteoid   The internal framework of bone without the mineral.

osteopenia   Means 'lack of bone', especially when viewed on an X-ray plate. Often used interchangeably with osteoporosis.

oxalate   From oxalic acid, the acid found in spinach and rhubarb, which binds calcium and makes it unavailable for absorption in the gut.

parathyroid glands   Four small glands in the neck which secrete parathyroid hormone.

parathyroid hormone   Sometimes shortened to parathormone. The hormone from the parathyroid which regulates the amount of calcium in the blood. Too much parathormone causes a high blood-calcium level, and an increased loss in the urine of calcium which has to come from the bones.

phytates   From phytic acids. Plant acids which can bind calcium and make it unavailable for absorption in the gut. They occur in cereals such as wheat, oats and rye. They are destroyed by the baker's-yeast enzymes in bread-making, but are not destroyed in unleavened bread or porridge.

pituitary gland   A small gland in the centre of the skull which makes hormones which influence other glands. Amongst these are follicle stimulating hormone, which stimulates the growth of the follicle in the ovary and the release of oestrogens; and luteinising hormone, which causes the follicle to release progestogens.

progestogens   Female hormones which build up the lining of the womb ready to receive a fertilised egg. If no fertilised egg appears, progestogens stop being made, and the lining of the womb is shed, i.e. menstruation.

prolactin   The hormone made by certain cells in the pituitary gland, which makes the breasts secrete milk. A tumour of these cells is called a prolactinoma and is a rare cause of osteoporosis.

radius   One of the bones in the forearm; the one on the thumb side.

receptor   A feature of a cell surface which allows a circulating hormone to attach itself to the cell. Without the appropriate receptor, the hormone cannot influence the cell. Receptors for oestrogens exist in many tissues apart from the breast, uterus and ovaries, including the skin, muscles and nervous system, and have recently been discovered in bone. This may be why oestrogen treatment affects many tissues other than just the female sex organs.

resorption   To resorb literally means to absorb back again. In the context of osteoporosis, resorption refers to the dissolving of bone by the osteoclasts.

rickets   Osteomalacia in the growing child.

scoliosis   An S-bend, from side to side, in the spine.

secondary deposits   The spread of cancer in tissues other than the one in which it started. Secondary deposits (or secondary growths) in bone commonly come from breast cancer, prostate cancer or lung cancer.

single-photon absorptiometry   Absorptiometry using radiation of one wavelength only.

thyroid gland   A gland in the front of the neck which produces two hormones which affect bone – calcitonin and thyroxin.

thyroxin   One of the hormones produced by the thyroid gland. Excess thyroxin speeds up all the body's processes, including the building up and resorption of bone. Unfortunately the resorption outpaces the building up, and osteoporosis results.

thyrotoxic osteoporosis   Osteoporosis resulting from excess thyroxin production from the thyroid gland.

ulna   The inner of the two bones in the forearm (the lower arm), on the little-finger side of the arm.

ultrasound Very high-pitched sound waves (so high you can't hear them) with an extremely short wavelength. Ultrasound is absorbed more by dense bones than by less dense osteoporotic bones. This has been used as one way of measuring osteoporosis.

uterus The womb.

vitamins Essential nutrients needed in trace amounts. They act as co-enzymes or necessary partners in many of the body's chemical changes.

USEFUL ADDRESSES

National Osteoporosis Society
Barton Mead House
PO Box 10
Radstock
Bath BA3 3YB
(0761) 32472

Age Concern (Head Office)
Bernard Sunley House
60 Pitcairn Road
Mitcham
Surrey CR4 3LL
(01) 640-5431

Age Concern Ireland
6 Lower Crescent
Belfast BT7 1NR
(0232) 245729

Age Concern Scotland
33 Castle Street
Edinburgh EH2 3DN
(031) 225-5000

Age Concern Wales
4th Floor
1 Cathedral Road
Cardiff CF1 9SD
(0222) 371821/371566

British Association of Occupational Therapists
20 Rede Place
London W2 4TU
(01) 229-9738

Brittle Bone Society (for Osteogenesis Imperfecta)
112 City Road
Dundee DD2 2PW
(0382) 67603

Dial UK (The National Association of Disablement Information and Advice Lines)
117 High Street
Clay Cross
Chesterfield
Derbyshire S45 9DZ
(0246) 250055

Disabled Living Centre Council
c/o Secretary of the Joint Aid Centres Council
76 Clarendon Park Road
Leicester LE2 3AQ
(0533) 700747

Disabled Living Foundation
380–384 Harrow Road
London W9 2HU
(01) 289-6111

Medic-Alert Foundation
11–13 Clifton Terrace
London N4 3JP
(01) 263-8596

National Council for Carers and their Elderly Dependents
29 Chilworth Mews
London WR2 3RG
(01) 262-1451

Royal Association for Disability and Rehabilitation
(RADAR)
25 Mortimer Street
London W1N 8AB
(01) 637-5400

Scottish Council on Disability
Princess House
5 Shandwick Place
Edinburgh EH2 4RG
(031) 229-8632

NORTH AMERICA

National Osteoporosis Foundation
1625 Eye Street NW, Suite 1011
Washington, DC 20006,
USA

Osteoporosis Society of Canada
76 St. Clair Avenue West
Toronto, Ontario M4V 1N2
Canada

INDEX

151